26 *days*

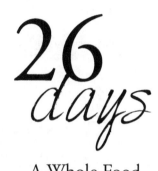

26 days

A Whole Food
Plant-Based Diet
and What You
Need to Know

CLAUDIA NICOLE

New York

26 *days*

A Whole Food Plant-Based Diet and What You Need to Know

Published in New York, New York, by Morgan James Publishing. Morgan James and The Entrepreneurial Publisher are trademarks of Morgan James, LLC. www.MorganJamesPublishing.com

The Morgan James Speakers Group can bring authors to your live event. For more information or to book an event visit The Morgan James Speakers Group at www.TheMorganJamesSpeakersGroup.com.

Shelfie

A **free** eBook edition is available with the purchase of this print book.

CLEARLY PRINT YOUR NAME ABOVE IN UPPER CASE

Instructions to claim your free eBook edition:
1. Download the Shelfie app for Android or iOS
2. Write your name in **UPPER CASE** above
3. Use the Shelfie app to submit a photo
4. Download your eBook to any device

ISBN 978-1-68350-049-0 paperback
ISBN 978-1-68350-050-6 eBook
ISBN 978-1-68350-051-3 hardcover
Library of Congress Control Number: 2016906531

Cover Design by:
Rachel Lopez
www.r2cdesign.com

Interior Design by:
Bonnie Bushman
The Whole Caboodle Graphic Design

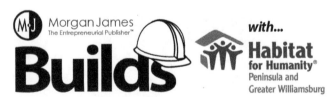

In an effort to support local communities, raise awareness and funds, Morgan James Publishing donates a percentage of all book sales for the life of each book to Habitat for Humanity Peninsula and Greater Williamsburg.

Get involved today! Visit www.MorganJamesBuilds.com

This book is for Lena, whom I love deeply and who inspires me to no end.

Table of Contents

According to the documentary *Forks Over Knives*, a whole food, plant-based diet is "a **diet based** on fruits, vegetables, tubers, **whole** grains, and legumes; and it excludes or minimizes meat (including chicken and fish), dairy products, and eggs, as well as highly refined **foods** like bleached flour, refined sugar, and oil."[1]

---

1   This definition was taken from the *Forks Over Knives* website: www.ForksOverKnives.com under "The FOK Diet."

Preface

I'm not an expert, nutritionist, doctor, facilitator, nor do I even consider myself athletic or in shape. I am someone who has just been concerned for years with what I eat; trying to make sense of the information I read and hear. After starting to write a journal on our daily eating habits, I realized there was a lot of truth in what I was thinking, doing, and reacting to. A journal can reveal a lot about the way we eat. The first part of this book is the first 26 days of my journal. There isn't a lot to discover other than how you might see yourself in my journal.

The second part of the book is what I call "my findings" which are my personal discoveries that I came to a conclusion on. And it's not just my own but my husband's experience too, as I write a lot about our conversations, our differences in the way we eat, and the choices we really tried to make together.

The next part of the book is what I have to say about this journey three months later. It's when this experiment has transformed interesting habits and with research, these habits grabbed my attention. It turns out that if I were to write an editorial, an op-ed article for a major newspaper or even a thesis, I would imagine having enough information from these studies to probably prepare something worthwhile. However, what I have chosen to do is publish this work and instead, create food for thought for the average reader.

The last section includes very simple, and what I consider, transitional plant-based recipes. When I was asked to create a few, I came up with almost forty-five. These are very common if not basic recipes for those who have probably never thought about this type of diet until now.

I had to pay my own way through college and although it's much harder to do so now, the information I can gather from experience combined with the Internet and Amazon could be the basis of an experimental study. The problem with our food habits is not so much an issue of choice but of culture and this is what I'd like to explain in this book. We are all guilty. Every single one of us. We are either on one extreme or the other while "middle America," people who are just trying to make better diet choices one day at a time, are consumed with having to make bad choices every day.

As it turns out, we all have one thing in common. We all like to eat. Everyone will be able to relate to my experience in trying to eat healthier. It is extremely painful to see people you love eat foods that extremists talk about as being poison and which we're sure to die from. My suggestion to all of you with these judgments is to stop immediately. This extreme way of thinking is not doing anyone any good.

What I discovered in writing this book is that we are not very different from each other. As I began to experiment with different recipes, talk to friends and family, read healthy articles, and watch documentaries, the answer is a lot simpler than all the radical information I can get my hands on. I have years of experience of meeting many different people with many different jobs and I can tell you, diet and health has been one of the most talked about conversations. I've not only had an interest in health, I find I'm no different from anyone reading this book. We are all actually alike.

This book is not to make claims, change laws, or promote anything different from what your medical doctors tell you. The information that I used and reference are not scientific and can't be proven because nothing can be absolutely proven. If I were to get the highest standards of research based on nutrition, there will still be a naysayer to argue against it. So what's the point?

Read this book without your filters and what you know. Take it in like you would a movie with a plot because that's all this is. I'm simply sharing a journey that turns out to be the hardest for many people. My only desire is to share with others an experience so that we can all look at each other and realize that our health, our diet, and our choices are all similarly difficult. No one has it easy. I am learning to be a better cook, a better wife, and a more compassionate aunt, sister, daughter, and friend after writing this book.

For all of you who want to eat better but are given such mixed messages with so many different diets to choose from, you're not alone. If I can get enough people to think before they eat and judge, I've accomplished a goal. My goal is not to get people to eat better but for us to start the conversation and realize no single person has the right answer. I would absolutely love for you to read my book and share with others. Thank you for reading it.

Acknowledgments

It's amazing how we meet people these days. Never would I have imagined meeting someone on Twitter that led to an invitation to attend a conference, to meeting him in person, to actually submitting a manuscript for review. As an exercise I completed that was only to be done to accomplish a goal, I submitted a manuscript for publication and before I realized it, I was working on a book for publication. It was happening.

If it wasn't for the countless people on social media who are trying to connect, grow their businesses, and share their ideas with the world, I would still be thinking about doing something like this like the countless other times, like the countless amount of people who do. I commend those on social media working towards their goals. One of them is Terry Whalin with Morgan James Publishing who has become a true soldier in finding people like me who just want to share their ideas. I'd like to thank him dearly for responding so quickly to all my questions.

I am blessed with an educated dad who has always taught me to know the meaning of words and a very street-smart mother who always told me that I can do anything I put my energy into. These two people have one thing in common:

they love their children. My hope is that their message comes out in this book as they both have taught me the balance between education and love.

And as you will soon know, this is not only my journey but my husband Richard's too. Most authors will thank their spouses for their support, but I have to say that my husband is more than a support. Richard has never opposed my sharing not only my journey but his as well. He has always supported every endeavor I've had especially when it includes him! It is true that I would not have been able to write this book without his unconditional support, but who else could I have talked about if not him? He is my friend, my confidant, my husband, and the love of my life. I thank him from the bottom of my heart.

Introduction

Are there dishes in your cabinet you never use? Do you eat leftovers the next day or do you put them in the fridge, only to throw them out when they're bad? Are the people you live with not supportive of your dieting? Is going to the grocery store boring? Do you ever research what you eat only to find what you're eating has harmful additives and find yourself confused? Do you want to change your diet but hate to fail over and over again? Is wine part of a plant-based wholesome diet?

It's my first day attempting to go without meat or dairy and the thoughts, attitudes, and opinions are shared with you. Little do I know that in a short period of time I would find out trying to follow this diet is much harder that I thought and there's a reason for this. There are ups and downs, but let me show you what happened when I incorporated a wholesome diet in our home. The first few weeks I struggled a little, but you need to know a few things before you start. The more you try, the better you'll get. But what if you knew things I found out here that could help you learn from my mistakes and move along faster?

It's not the same when I watch documentaries on my own and then try to incorporate the change by what I learn. A friend of mine told me to watch a documentary called *Forks Over Knives* after we had talked about healthy foods.

So I had my husband watch it with me. Yes, he was falling asleep at times. But as I became surprised, enraged, and confused, I was also inspired. I would nudge him to show him what I was seeing until he woke up and kept watching with me. He too became baffled. We've watched other documentaries in the past like *Food Inc.* so we were open to the concept.

We watched the *Forks Over Knives* documentary with Dr. Caldwell B. Esselstyn Jr. MD and Dr. T. Colin Campbell PhD reporting their studies and found them compelling. It still wasn't enough, though, to stop us from eating meat. But something happened. We watched it again at my sister's house. After casually watching these documentaries and studies over time, it was as if a light bulb went off. We were left with very few if any doubts, as were a lot of other people. It started to make sense. This documentary was about how Dr. T. Collin Campbell joined with China in one of the most ambitious studies on cancer from an atlas that was created showing cancer rates throughout China in more than 2,400 Chinese counties across China. Together with world-class scientists, Dr. Campbell pulled this team together and created The China Study, the most comprehensive study on cancer there is. They began a study that originated with over 650,000 workers who originated the atlas to a team of scientists, including the best epidemiologist in the world, to continue this research on health and diet that this atlas provided. Not many studies consist of this much research. "We had a study that was unmatched in terms of comprehensiveness, quality, and uniqueness."[2] In the documentary *Forks Over Knives*, the study consisted of helping a dozen patients get off their diabetes medication and they wanted to share their findings with the world.

We know it's not normal to see so many people around us who look as if they're tucking pillows down their clothes or are out of breath. Something is wrong when chairs are getting larger and doorways are being expanded. Open living spaces are becoming more common in our culture because we just don't fit into the confines of our doorways anymore. It's nice to think we're living differently, but let's look at how we are. Has it become no longer normal to separate entertainment from sitting at the dinner table?

---

2   When the study was done, there were more than 8,000 associations of significance according to *The China Study* by Dr. T. Colin Campbell PhD and Dr. Thomas M. Campbell MD, the producers of the *Forks Over Knives* documentary.

I feel as if I'm in a movie noticing that something strange is happening while everyone is oblivious to this scene as they ask for bigger chairs and wonder why the TV is not in the same room where they eat their dinner. Far be it for us to question this because we don't want to offend anyone else's "rights." So instead, I take on this challenge by attempting to document our first four weeks of adopting a new way of eating. One of the most important activities for any work of improvement, whether it's with your diet, spiritual growth, career, or anything, is to journal. A journal can reveal a lot.

Through keeping a journal, I learned that what we eat and how we feel affects our attitudes in all areas of our lives. After all, it's not a diet as much as an understanding of what we are doing to ourselves, right? Who hasn't heard, "you are what you eat?" By writing a journal, I find that trying to eat differently changes what we believe and that what we do expresses our true convictions—not necessarily what we say we believe. And isn't this what we try to find out through our journals?

We are taught what to eat all the time. "Don't eat this—eat that." And then that becomes bad too. Eggs were a major part of our diet and then they were too high in cholesterol. Now they're safe again. But in the past fifty years something has thrown us off course and is now wreaking havoc in our lives, financially and physically. We don't feel well. We spend a lot of money on food. Restaurants have no limits on how much fat and calories they can add to their foods while ruining our diets in one sitting. Our time spent enjoying family and friends is combined with delicious food smothered in butter. At the same time, we are literally damaging our planet while people go hungry. Never mind the drugs prescribed to us for our ailments—that's for a different book. We buy green products, are proud to drive electric cars, and save on bags at the grocery store in an attempt to help revolutionize the earth. However, like everything else it starts in the home.

This journal attempts to bring you into our home to show you what I discover, to help people see what I see. (Do you see what I'm seeing? Would you be able to relate?) The truth is in how we live and it's in what we are feeding ourselves. If we can understand how we eat, together, we can help each other continue the attack on the fastest growing disease that is killing us: ignorance.

My husband and I don't have kids or regular day jobs, and some people may find this lifestyle is easier for us because of our circumstances. The challenge is all the same for most of us, though. At least with what I have discovered, we will all, without a doubt, be able to relate. I'm certainly not right all the time and don't dig into the information deep enough to help convince others. Keep in mind this is a journal.

My hope is that each of us will journal our own stories with our own experiences because they won't all be the same. But understanding what we have to change may somehow be the same for all of us. At least everyone can journal.

So here it is.

Part I

THE JOURNAL

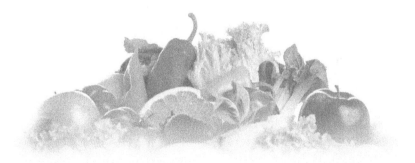

Chapter 1

The Grocery Store

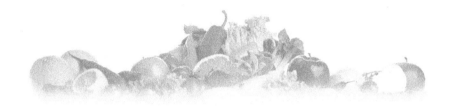

I take my usual walk around the circumference of the store. That's what the "experts" advise. By shopping only in the outer aisles and not the inside ones, I understand I will avoid a lot of processed foods and for the most part they were right. However, it was actually depressing as I strolled around the store. I passed the deli-carved meat station, the bread, the butter, the cheese, the meats, the eggs, and then the milk. This was going to be tougher than I thought. Our new way of eating was causing me to wonder if I was in the right store.

For the first time, I cut across the aisles and picked up some water. "Great! I can get that! Detergent for my hand washables—check!"

As I finally reached the produce department, I was free. Free to move about and out of "danger." I was sure others noticed my basket full of produce and probably thought I looked nothing like someone who ate only produce. Does she have cancer? I'm sure they wondered. Should I buy the caramel or fruit dips to help eat more fruit? No, they have too much sugar or additives. I would never think about a bag of expensive pistachios, but they were on sale. I toss those suckers in the basket—I'll need all the protein I can get—then keep moving. So what if I become some sort of chipmunk or squirrel? After grabbing cabbage, kale, tomatoes, squash, onions, Portabella mushrooms (what I would use to replace the steak), and garlic, I realized I could use beans for protein too.

I walk down the front of the aisles toward the front of the store when I stop in my tracks. What was I getting? I keep walking.

I pick up a gluten-free pizza in the frozen foods section on the way to where I was going even though I don't remember what it was and think, so what! I find some summer knick-knacks on sale on a table and fill the void of not buying anything I want by tossing these in the basket as well. I add a red mug from the Fourth of July stack and a mustard and ketchup set to put chocolate or caramel in for the desserts I'll desperately need after eating like this. I toss them in the basket.

I keep walking then realize I'll need something to eat with all this produce. Quinoa! I walk toward the back of the store, trying to remember dry, dry, dry foods. I find a newly packaged brand of red lentils, kidney beans, black beans, regular lentils, and quinoa. Great. These companies are always prepared for what I'm looking for. I grab them all as if they'll satisfy a hunger after days of food deprivation. I head toward the canned tomatoes section and buy a can of whole tomatoes. Then I realized the Asian aisle was around the corner. Asian food! Of course!

I find clear noodles, canned bamboo shoots, and bean sprouts, go for the Udon noodles but then decide to skip the pasta. I would select the dried seaweed snacks I've seen a friend feed her children but think that's going too far. At that moment I realized, probably a good forty-five minutes into my shopping, that, although I was grabbing at straws, I was opening up new dish ideas I had thought of preparing before but never did. I can add bamboo shoots to a dish that substituted for meat one time. (Just what was that dish?)

At this point, I thought I should make my way to the register. I'm surely over my budget with all this stuff I hardly ever buy; I knew my binge shopping had put me over the limit.

At the register, I'm amazed to find I'm well under my usual bill even though I had stocked up on a lot of stuff! Ka-ching!

At home, I make Portabella mushroom tacos[3] with onions, jalapenos, and tomatoes. I top them with cilantro, hot sauce, and Cotija cheese, a staple I always have in my fridge. (We're starting slowly.) I was full with just two tacos. I'm so happy Richard has decided to do this with me, and he liked the tacos. But then he said we'll be eating a lot of fish and chicken from now on. (What?) At least we were getting as close to a plant-based diet as possible. Then I realized it was okay to move ahead slowly. It was bad enough telling him the amount of milk he consumed did more harm than good, especially skim milk. I heard my acupuncturist say skim milk is much worse than one percent milk, and he was drinking almost a gallon a week. What did we know? I'm certain an acupuncturist would know more than the both of us put together.

---

3   This recipe is in the back of the book under "Dinner."

Chapter 2

He Drank the Almond Milk!

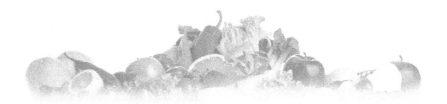

I made shakes this morning using a shake mix we don't like, but we've made a decision so we used it. It wasn't that bad. I used the bananas, which I won't worry about going bad anymore. I'll use the strawberries tomorrow.

I made coffee but realized halfway through the morning that I hadn't touched it. I made it through the morning, though. Richard didn't have lunch and neither did I. That probably wasn't a good idea because we were pretty hungry for dinner.

I decided to take out a bag of bean medley from the back of my pantry that had been there longer than I can remember, skipping all the bags of beans I'd just bought. I soaked the complete package of bean medley; not even thinking it might have been too much for two people. I know now to use more than half of the bag of whatever beans I use. Typically a bag or box of anything is hardly enough even for the two of us, except for pasta. I'm used to using half the bag or box of pasta.

Should I use the crockpot? It's about 10 a.m., so I decide to soak them in the crockpot for now. A few hours later, the beans had soaked up almost all the water. Wow!

At around 3 p.m., I put them in a pot and poured in some leftover stock and gluten-free bouillon that had been in the pantry for over a year. I normally use the regular bouillon but figured while I was at it I might as well use gluten-free. I used two cubes in case it wasn't as flavorful and added a little salt and a few garlic cloves, filled up the pot, and turned on the stove for it to boil. Back in my home office, I soon started to smell the wonderful aroma that penetrated the whole house.

Later, I chopped carrots, onions, and cabbage and reached for the chopped kale. Each went in according to how long it took, making it colorful. I also heated last night's Portabella mushrooms for tacos on the side. I didn't have avocados to top off as a relish, nor did I remember to use the cilantro I normally use. Instead, I reached for the lemons and squeezed some into the nine-bean medley soup[4]. I was in the zone.

Richard was adamant about going out for a run. He didn't have a major workout but seemed happy he went. I've been working late and haven't worked out for the past two days, but with our new diet, I'm not going to feel as bad today.

I would have had two bowls as I normally do, but I was full after one. I can get full pretty quickly with these kinds of vegetable soups. As they mentioned in *Forks Over Knives*, vegetables fill you up really well. It's true.

After one bowl for me and two for Richard, I still had a huge pot left over. I was able to pour the soup in four Ziploc bags and freeze them. I put them all in the freezer. They should be good for lunches or dinners.

For dessert, I brought out the canned pears I had stored in a plastic container in the fridge almost a week ago. I had put them in the fridge with the best intentions of having a better dessert, but after a few bites they were left in the fridge and forgotten. Now I can report that after dinner these were refreshing and thoroughly enjoyed. The next day, though, I don't think we had anything to celebrate yet.

---

4   I don't include the entire recipe but I write about it in the back of the book under "Dinner."

Chapter 3

One Notch Better Than a Bust

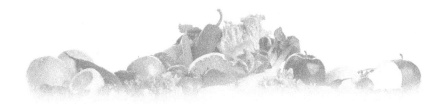

Ⓘt was tough, but we both managed to do a workout this morning. When I returned from mine Richard was eating his toast and jam. I reminded him he could have had it with peanut butter—his favorite PB and J.

I scrambled to figure out what to have for myself, but that had given me an idea. I had some delicious gluten-free bread with peanut butter and, you guessed it, bananas. I forgot the strawberries, though. I spread peanut butter on top of my gluten-free raisin bread, sliced the banana, and layered it on top. I had read that if you sprinkle sesame seeds on top you can add fiber, but I forgot to do that too.

For lunch, I threw out old pasta that was going bad in the refrigerator. I thought about having a salad but remembered my acupuncturist did not recommend I have cold foods for now, including salad—another food that is supposed to be good for me but isn't. Apparently, cold foods, including salads and cold protein shakes, were not good during treatment. I reached for the mozzarella instead, convincing myself I needed to get rid of it anyway, and melted it between the last two corn tortillas. If I couldn't have what I thought I needed, I was giving into warm cheese. I was about to go into a conference call for the morning so I had to make something fast. Now that I think about it, I should have put some spinach on it.

Although the acupuncturist had also told me how harmful it was to go through a whole gallon of milk in one week, I decided to deplete all our meat and dairy products instead of throwing them out while people on this planet went hungry. I would no longer buy meat and dairy products and instead replace them with fruits, vegetables, beans, and whole grain foods. Seeing an acupuncturist had been my last resort. My regular doctor informed me of a condition I had that was most likely going to put me on medication indefinitely. I was not comfortable taking medication, let alone indefinitely. Plus, having uncomfortable testing done is the reason I thought I would try an acupuncturist.

It turned out we both blew it for lunch. Richard admitted he had KFC for lunch and even got the original recipe with mashed potatoes, coleslaw, and a biscuit. I suppose this was his way of eating healthier than the pizza or hot dog from Costco. I guess I should be supportive of his trying at least.

We both had to be at a meeting later that evening, but we didn't have time to grab dinner except to take it with us. Should we get a chicken burrito and split it? We ended up splitting a rotisserie chicken plate with vegetables and coleslaw. At least we didn't overeat.

We confirmed to have dinner with friends this weekend; the challenge would be finding a place. They asked if we would like to have pork bellies at a great Korean BBQ restaurant in Korea Town in Los Angeles. I confessed to my friend that we were trying to abstain from meat and dairy for a month. Ugh. Okay, I would have to think of something good.

With that, today was one notch better than a bust. It was certainly better than what we normally ate. When we got home from our meeting, we finished the pears and were content. But I wasn't convinced we were making the decisions we needed to make.

Chapter 4

Decisions, Decisions

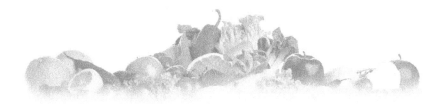

This morning I didn't forget the strawberries. I put them in a shake with aloe vera juice, ice, and protein powder with strawberry flavoring from another shake brand we liked. Not all protein powders are made equal. Some are fantastic while others are gross. The challenge was finding a good one that tasted better and was somewhat good for you. I discovered some were neither. I didn't add the chia seeds this time to ensure it had a smooth consistency to keep the momentum going with Richard. And it worked. He said it was the best one yet even though I knew it still wasn't as good as our old shake brand.

Then I made coffee.

I didn't go to the gym this morning so I went during lunch and ran hard. I weighed myself afterward and was less than 140 pounds, at 139.6. I'd been weighing from 143 to 148 pounds for weeks, so that was encouraging. It was still a far cry from my average of 128, but I accepted 139 for now.

I got home and, after rummaging through the fridge, I decided to eat a quesadilla but with spinach. Even though the pepper jack was staring at me and I knew it would have been perfect, I chose a .17 ounce of specialty soft white cheese I had originally bought to eat with wine. Maybe it was made with better ingredients than the jack cheese, but who was I kidding? I was simply eating a very good cheese I hated to let go to waste. Yes, that was probably more of the truth. And with it being so small, I added only a few pieces and had a quesadilla made primarily of spinach. The cheese served as a glue to make the spinach stick. Maybe this would lessen the blow of knowing it was a flour tortilla instead of the corn tortillas we were out of. I added a few strawberries on the side, poured myself a sparkling water and felt as if this was a lunch on any other diet program. I was cheating, though, by adding the cheese delicacy.

I like sparkling water. When I went to Europe, they would ask if I wanted it flat or with fizz. I don't care for flat water and am not someone to drink much water anyway, but I recently found out I can drink a lot of sparkling water. I think about all those people like me who don't drink water and struggle not to have soda all the time. Well, the Europeans have it figured out. Either you like sparkling water or flat water. If you don't like flat water, you're probably a sparkling water drinker. Don't like it plain? Just find out which juice or flavoring you'll drink with it. Maybe I'll get that appliance that makes homemade sparkling water.

Richard had chicken linguini for lunch. He hasn't graduated to having a plant-based meal yet, but it was also something he wouldn't have had for lunch before we decided to change our diet (even though the reality of our decision isn't quite there yet). He seemed to be scrambling around too. He said it was just a little portion. Well, it isn't going to happen overnight.

For dinner we had another meeting to attend, so Richard picked up some Panda Express. I told him to order rice and vegetables for me. He had his usual orange chicken, but this time with broccoli. I'd always told him he should have at least a vegetable with his orange chicken, but he would refuse. He didn't need to add that, but now it's different. I didn't think we were doing well at all, but at least he was being more mindful of eating vegetables and making better decisions. He would never have ordered vegetables before with orange chicken.

Everything I read is always about making drastic decisions from steak to vegetables in a day. This has got to be the toughest decision for a lot of people. My grandmother stopped smoking by just making that decision but not all people can do that. What most of us can do is adapt.

The next night was the Korean BBQ dinner we planned with friends and I was hoping I could just have soup. We would see.

Chapter 5

Not Really the Last of the Meat

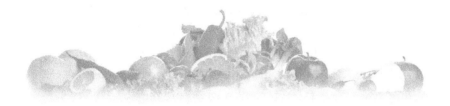

In the morning we had toast. Richard found it easy to fix toast with jelly. It wasn't the best breakfast, but I reminded myself that we're working slowly. I like avocado and had slices on my toast. I have a great chili lime spice I like to drizzle on it, either over toast or a corn tortilla, and it's delicious. Richard isn't there yet, although I'm not sure what the big deal is about having avocado on toast. He'll have guacamole but not avocado slices because he says it's like eating slices of butter.

Many of us have these psychological memes, a cultural impression in our minds that is repeated in a manner comparable to the transmission of genes. This is the effect memes can have. This is how our abilities and even willingness to eat healthy is challenged. Nevertheless, as I'm writing this, guacamole it is. I'll smash the avocado and spread "guacamole" on his toast. We'll just see how that goes.

I struggled with deciding whether to take the cheese we had left out of the fridge—the cheese I'd decided to phase out. We had a whole brick of pepper jack cheese and half a cheddar block I used for making quesadillas. It's the quickest snack I've known for as long as I can remember. Not grabbing the cheese might be as hard as any temptation there is. Habits like these are the toughest challenge, especially if you've been doing it almost since the beginning of your time on earth. I have yet to figure out what I'm going to do with the cheese, but I can't let it go to waste. If I were diabetic and the doctor told me to make this radical change literally overnight, I guess I would have to, but I'm the only one who'll benefit by doing this now. Not to mention, with all the starving children in the world . . . All of a sudden, I felt a sense of logic kick in.

As we're working to figure this out and find enough foods we can eat, I couldn't help but decide to have the ground lamb I bought about a week and a half ago. I bought it before we decided to venture into a world of no meat and dairy although Richard is still convinced he can have chicken and fish. The verdict is out with me, though. I think I can do fine without meat at all.

Having lamb was about the extent of cheating for the day. I had coffee with my friend who said she had the steak, the bread, the pasta, and the dessert before she finally felt guilty and this was after a week-long binge of eating out all week for her birthday. I think because we made this decision, allowing one item to ruin our lifestyle was enough for us to feel guilty. How many times have I been in that position of guilt after days of indulging myself? Too many to count. I start to wonder what this does to oneself—the repeated feelings of guilt.

I went to the store to pick up a few veggies and coconut oil. That's all I needed. But I also picked up fish, sauces, and two mini-size crab cakes. I thought one crab cake with a white wine would be our reward. I started to look at the packaging on items to see what ingredients were in sauces, frozen foods, and even vinegar! Yes, vinegar. I found coconut vinegar. I didn't know they made something like that.

I made the spaghetti squash I had sitting on the counter for over a week. I looked over a few recipes on Google, thought about it for a while, and decided to make ground lamb with onions, tomatoes and cilantro, and a bruschetta sauce. I scraped the squash out of the shell and what do I know? It looked like spaghetti. I served the lamb over the spaghetti squash. It was delicious! Richard said the squash was tasty although to him it *felt like* eating waxed string. It's funny how we eat based on what we're used to psychologically. It's no wonder I felt disappointed the next day. Although it was delicious, it's not the same if your spouse doesn't think it's just as good.

Chapter 6

Disappointed

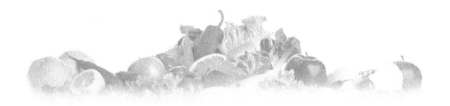

O kay, this day wasn't the easiest. I went to a morning breakfast meeting and the only item I can order on the menu is oatmeal. It's one of the few items besides coffee I could have. I'll pour creamer into it to make it creamier because I hate dry-tasting oatmeal. That's what I'm used to. I was pouring it in when I realized I was messing up again. I didn't opt for the coffee this time. I ordered a green tea with honey. Surprisingly, I ended up not even finishing the oatmeal. I ate maybe two-thirds of it and wondered if my subconscious was kicking in. Or was it the tea? So far, having a plant-based breakfast is challenging.

I was pretty full for most of the day. It wasn't until around 3 p.m. that I felt famished. Great. Now what?

I went for the traditional healthy green apple and peanut butter snack. I'll typically have only half the apple when snacking, but this time I couldn't get enough of it. I took the whole jar of peanut butter with my sliced apple to my desk and devoured the whole apple with the help of the peanut butter. That was my lunch.

Dinner was a different story. Tonight we were going to have Korean BBQ to celebrate my friend's birthday. I'd thought I would cook the chicken I'd found in the freezer. I figured we could eat it before we left. That way, with all that "protein" we would eat before going for Korean BBQ, we could order something like a vegetable soup and be okay. From what I've always heard, meat as a protein keeps you from being hungry for longer periods of time. But that's not what happened. Richard was not coming home until around 7 p.m. I shut down my computer around 5:30 p.m., realizing I hadn't picked up a card and gift for my friend for her birthday.

I ran out and was lucky to be able to find something quickly and got back close to 7 p.m. when Richard came home. Our friends were scheduled to pick us up soon. Fortunately for us, they picked us up late and we were able to shower and meet them downstairs. So much for the chicken and the idea of proving to our friends how disciplined we were.

The spot for dinner was a small bar in Korea Town and it was fantastic. My Korean friend navigated her way around to help us order. It was funny to have to check online for all the pictures so we could see what we were ordering. Forget trying to figure out what was in each dish. The choices were pork ribs, calamari, soup, cooked rice cakes in a spicy sauce, spicy chicken, and a delicious eel wrap that turned out to be very good. The eel wrap was the only dish that had any hint of vegetables. Our friends were willing to work with us and not have any meat, but Richard couldn't help himself and ordered the pork ribs as the final order. I think our friends were surprised too after we boldly told them about our new way of eating. Richard said it was a special occasion. Really?

Was it worth ordering the ribs? No, it wasn't. My friend's Korean ribs were better. Hers are more tender and flavorful and what we had to compare with ribs in a Korean BBQ restaurant. That's like comparing a home-cooked meal to something you order in a bar, but the idea of having an excuse to eat meat was blinding our assertions. The feel of a cool place changed to sort of a letdown; we ordered the pork ribs thinking this would have been well worth us cheating, but once again it wasn't. It turned out to be a gamble and our disappointment was our loss. We ate through the dish with everyone having a few nibbles without completely devouring it. It was good, but we were both disappointed in ourselves. We talked about it on the way home. Was this enough to restart the whole plan?

Chapter 7

Saturday Reboot

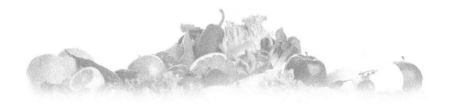

I was out the door at 8 a.m. but not before having almost the last of the Fage, my favorite plain Greek yogurt. I knew that when the yogurt was gone it would be gone for a very long time, so I enjoyed it as much as I could.

I headed to the gym and Richard went for a run. As I walked to the gym, I knew I needed coffee but the thought of having even a small cup seemed a lot as I was still feeling the BBQ ribs settling in my stomach. So, this morning, I went for a single shot of espresso at Coffee Bean on my way to the gym. When I was given the espresso from the barista, I headed to the milk station out of habit but I sipped it without wanting any milk in it. I was drinking it to wake up, not for comfort. I did enough of that last night. I drank the espresso quickly and headed to the gym. Why hadn't I ever thought about that? Having just a single shot without the milk was not such a bad idea. I was still satisfied.

My workout was good. I not only got on the bike but had enough energy to run on the treadmill too. I didn't think I'd accomplish that, but I did, thanks to the straight-up coffee. I think my workouts are getting better. I think.

I didn't have much time to make breakfast because we had no pancake mix and no eggs. I told Richard eggs were dairy and he couldn't have those either. He moaned. I tried to get him to have peanut butter with bananas in a tortilla, but that didn't pass. I cut melon and strawberries and we had that. I knew that wasn't going to be enough, though. I told him I'd make breakfast if he stayed home today and didn't go into the office, but now I didn't know what to make for breakfast.

I thought about making chicken sausages with peppers and onions as I typically make on a "diet," but now sausages were not an option. I once again rummaged through the fridge and found one last vegan hot dog—my attempt at being a wannabe vegan. This was when I came up with slicing the hot dog with peppers and onions. So I thought, here goes nothing. I sautéed the sliced vegan hot dog in coconut oil with peppers and onions and then added garlic powder at the end. I was determined to get him to like this. I served it as if it was no big deal and off he went into another room, taking the dish with him.

I made myself toast with gluten-free bread, peanut butter, and sliced bananas. I remembered buying different types of nut butter. I should really get those out and mix it up! Richard came back out with an empty plate. He mumbled something and, just when I was about to argue back, he said it was good! Wow. Really?

I mixed a "green" chocolate-flavored mix in almond milk but didn't like it. I was going to drink it, but after coming back to it the second time I decided to toss it. It was kind of gross. I then spent the next hour or so clearing out my spice shelves.

We ran errands all afternoon. When we came home, we opened a bottle of pinot and had it with appetizers. I chopped tomatoes, cucumber, and tarragon and mixed everything with olive oil even though the oil didn't qualify as being on a plant-based diet. We had this spread[5] with rice crackers. Instead of having just cheese as we normally do, I chopped tiny pieces of the .17 ounce goat cheese

---

5   I include this simple recipe in the back of the book under "Appetizers."

I had bought to have with wine and tossed it with canned beets I also chopped. Richard doesn't like beets, but he apparently liked them chopped up with the cheese sprinkled with tarragon. Amazing! As long as he didn't ask me what it was we were good. I finished baking the chicken I'd covered with spices and onions and sautéed cabbage, kale, garlic, and dried cranberries. Cranberries are my favorite dollar-store find. Richard typically picks them out, but apparently he ate the whole thing, even the cranberries this time. As I document this, I notice these things even more.

For dessert, we had sliced strawberries sautéed in port and a squirt of whipped cream—another dairy product we're finishing before it's totally gone. We were done. So much for the reboot.

Chapter 8

Changing It Up a Bit

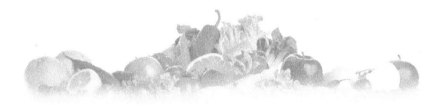

We changed things up a bit today. We typically go to my sister's on Sunday evenings for our weekly family dinner get-together and have smoked ribs, hamburgers, hot dogs, sausages, and tons of carbs. It's delicious. Then, as if that's not enough, we have pie, chocolate cake, or another decadent dessert, but not before having a few bottles of Napa's finest.

Today, however, we decided to stay home and continue working on this new way of eating. Besides, we felt great about finishing a huge project yesterday when we ran errands and wanted to keep that momentum going today. We were a bit drained from all the meetings of the week anyway and driving sixty miles today to see family didn't sound too appealing. The momentum seemed to stem from being on a mission.

We had fruit in the morning before heading to church and I had coffee. The option to stop for a croissant or donut was out of the question and although we were running a little late, we didn't even talk about it. I knew it was on his mind, though, as much as it was on mine. We kept quiet on the way to church.

We met with friends after church for lunch. We hesitated but agreed. What was surprising was that, although Richard was not ever into eating at Chipotle, he agreed to go there. I like Chipotle. I've always liked the organic fast food options they have, like their famous lime rice with cilantro and the tacos that make a good fast food meal. This time, however, I noticed they had what you call "sofritas," a crumbled type of tofu that was seasoned with spices and chili sauce, and I was willing to try it. It was not only delicious, but I learned a new way of making tofu. Richard went for his usual chicken burrito. I saw him ask for the cheese and sour cream and then look at me with disappointment; without my asking, he said he forgot.

What was interesting was that after lunch we were determined to get more stuff done. We ran more errands although it felt like a lazy Sunday afternoon. We got home, relaxed, and enjoyed our favorite Sunday night TV show. I opened a bottle of wine and Richard went for a run.

For appetizers, I brought out the leftover-diced tomatoes and cucumber with tarragon, beets and goat cheese, and rice crackers. It was very nice and as much a luxury as it was eating sausage and cheese by itself. Most of the time, if I'm honest with myself, as much as the summer sausage tastes good, I've always known it wasn't the best thing for us to eat.

I blew it on dinner, though; somehow I forgot how to cook green beans. I made salmon with green beans. Pretty simple, but I forgot to steam the green beans before sautéing them with garlic. We ate the salmon I had seasoned with spices instead of salt and pepper. If we're going to have meat, I might as well cut back on the salt. It wasn't bad, but the green beans were not cooked. I know to steam green beans before sautéing them, but I guess it had been so long since I've had them. I did imagine the ham, bacon bits, and prosciutto it needed for a dash of grease, but they were not cooked and no amount of meat would have made them taste better.

We were so discouraged from trying to eat right today. I steamed the green beans later and put them in the fridge. We were over it today. How much more disappointment and torture can we take?

Chapter 9

Monday Strike-Out

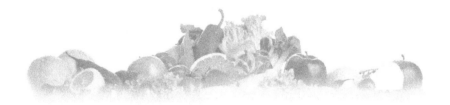

I got up and went to the gym. I continued my routine of riding the bike and that was fine. It was as good a workout as it could be for a Monday. I succumbed to my usual café 'ole which is half steamed milk and half coffee but for some reason it didn't taste as good today. Maybe I should have stuck to my espresso.

I made a fruit smoothie for Richard when I got back. I'm like the lead chef around here, trying to control our home menu and keep it as whole food, plant-based as I can although I'm not doing a great job of it. So, with that, I went ahead and put the chia seeds into the shake mix this time with about four ounces of orange juice and an equal amount of coconut milk. Halfway through drinking my shake I wondered if I should have put in honey, but it tasted fine. With all the fruit and orange juice it had about as much sugar as anyone needed. I felt pretty good about that, took my share of it, gave the other part to Richard, and walked back to my office. I then heard the toaster and the jar of homemade jam open from my office. He was having strawberry jam on toast. I guess sharing the shake wasn't enough for Richard.

I went back to the kitchen and made some tea and toast. I was hungry too and realized it was probably because we were left short-changed last night. I not only had peanut butter on my toast but also maple-flavored almond butter. I thought having different flavors of peanut butter could do the trick, but it didn't. The different flavors tasted like peanut butter.

I came home after a late afternoon appointment and Richard came home shortly afterward. I realized I hadn't had any lunch and Richard was probably hungry too. I had taken out some bean soup to thaw for lunch and offered some to Richard; he gave me a face that didn't look very appeased. I heated it anyway and added hot sauce—everything is good with hot sauce, right? Poor thing ate as much as he could. Fortunately, I had some gluten-free pizza to give him from the freezer so I heated it in the toaster and of course the temperature was wrong; he bit into a cold bread roll to boot.

I told him I had the last of the meat left which was the ground lamb I had in the freezer. I'm not sure why I froze it; maybe because we love lamb so much. I told him that to try to make up for the awful stuff I was bringing out. I was doing as much as I could, but I was striking out left and right.

Later, he left for an appointment and I went back to work. When he came home I'm sure he was expecting food on the stove, but none was there. He went out for a run and I decided to make enchiladas and spinach. The lamb was still a bit frozen, so I had to make something different quickly if I was going to continue having any influence on him.

Dinner was good and I finished the last of the Fage yogurt that substituted for sour cream. Funny how I would usually feel good about having this as a substitute, but today I need to finish it for good—or at least a very long time.

After dinner, I reached for the chocolate mint cookies. I settled for having a few nibbles on a broken cookie. That was good enough. I gave one cookie to Richard and he was overjoyed. I'm not sure it prepared me for what I would put myself through on the weekend, though.

Chapter 10

Ready to End It

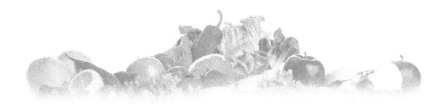

I don't know if I was giving in from the get-go, but I was in the mood for something simple. I went to a breakfast meeting this morning. I hardly ever have pancakes, but today I felt like having them. There was no meat or dairy in them, except for the melted butter that was an absolute must. And since I'm talking about a must have, I went ahead with the butter.

On my way out of the restaurant, I was just about to pass the deli with baked goods by the front door before I decided to pick up a cherry turnover for my sister who I was traveling to San Diego for the weekend with. She loves those and what's not to love? They're really delicious here. Of course, they're never available except today when I noticed the baker putting them in the display. In the spirit of good food and good camaraderie, I ordered it up and made great conversation with the baker behind the counter. My sister's going to love the surprise!

Today, I knew, was going to be a challenge. I'll be spending the weekend in San Diego for an overnight trip. My sister enjoys life, people, and a great steak and this weekend we're driving to San Diego to visit a friend who is in town; almost two hours away for the theater, drinks, and good food. Who's to argue with that? After breakfast, I took the train to meet her. She picked me up, we rented a car, and got on the road headed into San Diego. Of course, on our way down to San Diego from Orange County, she wanted to pick up lunch. Our absolute favorite is Der Wienerschnitzel. Now this is an institution for both of us, especially when we're together. Wienerschnitzel is just another way of bonding with my sister. Everyone has a vice and, for most of us, we enjoy them more when we are with family and friends. At one time, we put away at least six dogs with fries, a couple of sodas, and maybe a few corn dogs. It's just one of those things we like to do together. It isn't good for the body, but it is good for the relationship! So without guilt, I searched for the closest Wienerschnitzel off the freeway on my phone. I Googled "Wienerschnitzel locations. "

When we found one off the freeway, I ended up having my usual chilidog with onions and a hot-dog-on-a-stick combo. I would usually have this with milk to soothe my stomach from the chili, but I opted for a lime soda instead. I also ordered the 100 percent Angus beef dog, but the bun wasn't as soft. I tried.

After a few hours back on the road, we met her friends and had a cocktail. We then headed to the restaurant—a Mexican restaurant. I'm done! I thought. I was going to be completely out of commission today and let loose. I should forget this day altogether.

But something interesting happened.

We arrived at a fairly hip restaurant in San Diego and I saw not only "GF" and "VG" by a few of the menu items but also "PB." Can it be? Only one entrée was plant-based and a few appetizers as well. How can I not order the only plant-based dish on the menu?

The cauliflower tacos were really good! I was full from two of the three tacos. I ordered a fancy Michelada too, which is typically beer mixed with lime juice and Clamato or tomato juice. This one, however, had a green salsa and lime juice. This sounded interesting so I had to try it. It wasn't bad but I was happier that they had something plant-based and good. I learned that guacamole glued everything together and it worked quite nicely. I asked for a doggie bag to take the last taco out of three. I can just pick on this in the car on the way home. I'm amazed at the thrills I get these days!

A theater show, nibbles of spectacular desserts in a specialty dessert restaurant with about eleven other people, a few more after-hour cocktails, and I was ready to end it.

I put the tacos and the turnovers in the mini fridge in our hotel. It was 2:30 a.m. and my head hit the pillow.

Chapter 11

Redemption

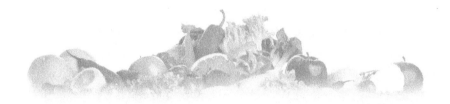

The morning wasn't so bad getting up. My sister and I were closing out the weekend by heading to the farmer's market. I didn't think too much about it other than that I was finally able to go. Richard doesn't like going to farmer's markets and we're always too busy on Saturdays or Sunday mornings anyway. The only actual farmer's market near us is the original farmer's market on Third and Fairfax in Los Angeles. This farmer's market is more of a landmark; it's a smorgasbord of different cultural foods and some produce. But to say this was a nearby farmer's market is like calling Disneyland a nearby park.

The weather was hot and the farmer's market in San Diego was extensive, stretching for about five to six blocks. Like finding a gluten-free section at Whole Foods for the first time, it was exciting to see the amount of whole food, plant-based items that were the majority rather than the minority.

They had vegetarian and vegan products like spreads, tamales, nuts, samosas, and Indian food. It was a food festival blitz! The great part was walking with my sister and pointing out all the goodness, all the wonderful plant-based choices. Never mind that a cherry turnover was still sitting in the car. Fruits and vegetables were lined up and the atmosphere was like going to a promotional event for a healthier lifestyle. Perfect! Where have I been? I've always known this about farmer's markets, but it was nice to be reminded why these markets are such a haven for the minority of eaters who have learned to eat healthier and create their own marketplace. My sister even talked about carrying a cooler with her on our next trip! (Cha-ching!)

After talking with friends about going vegan (never mind a plant-based diet), I've heard what people say about eating a healthier diet. Among them are: "I've known someone who tried it and it made her a meaner person," "My body is anemic and it tells me I need to eat meat," "As long as we exercise, we are fine." Listening to comments such as these from others is like being in the twilight zone with everyone saying how sugar is such a needed food because they crave it so much. It's like hearing zombies. But it's the lack of information that makes us zombies.

If the majority only internalized the studies, the research, and the countless years of research that have revealed that eating meat and dairy is linked to heart disease, diabetes, cancer, and other diseases, would eating primarily plant-based foods be as accepted as being Christian when we don't act like one? Sure, everyone wants to lose weight, but that's just the beginning. I've heard about people who lose weight by only eating meat as their source of needed protein. And they do! And I did too! We're also advancing clogged arteries and disease, which is great for the naysayers who are opposed to any diets or any changes, for that matter. No wonder we're all confused!

Acquiring a whole food, plant-based lifestyle hasn't made me lose weight right away, but I'm not gaining unnecessary fat either. When your blood pressure is lowered, your cholesterol reduced, and your sinuses cleared, your mind starts to work. You might gain clearer thinking that will help you to be more organized, more productive and, in turn, more active. It's the process, the road that leads to a skinnier version of you. At least this is what I'm finding for myself.

With that, we returned back home to my sister's house where Richard met us. For our weekend family dinner, we had mushrooms sautéed in Italian butter and balsamic vinegar and asparagus with pepper, lemon, and a basil olive oil, cooked together. The asparagus was also cooked with filet mignons rubbed in Cajun spices together in a smoker. I suggested the filets be sliced and served as appetizers instead of as an entrée, and my brother-in-law agreed! I had about two medium-rare slices that melted in my mouth. I was cheating and felt completely helpless.

Chapter 12

Church Day

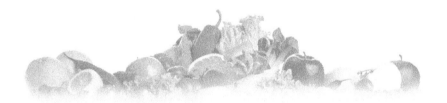

There's nothing a cup of coffee can't cure and I can always count on it at my sister's house. She has a single-cup brew maker, a ten-cup coffeemaker, an electric teakettle, and an assortment of sugars, creamers, hot chocolates, and other mixes on her countertop. A cup of coffee with the cherry turnover I traveled with all weekend was delicious even though it was just a sliver. My sister declined for the moment. It was Sunday morning at my sister's house and Richard and I were up and ready to head out as usual.

Richard and I drove to church. We participate in leading groups, watching kids, and sometimes helping in meetings before or right after the service. Today after church, we had a meeting and I was unprepared for it. I didn't realize we had one today. At these meetings lunch is usually served. I thought if we have sandwiches, I'd be done for—with submarine sandwiches and all the bread and meat that are supposed to be the healthier choice. A nice sandwich with a bag of chips is another one of my favorites. I would most likely give in to that, but it turned out it was El Pollo Loco with chicken, beans, rice, and salad. Perfect!

I did pick up a very small drumstick and cheated on that. Maybe it was the abundance of grilled chicken in two large bowls that got me. Regardless, I was without control on the chicken. Maybe if we were more prepared with our calendar I would have made our own lunch like some others do on their diets. Anyway, I poured the beans over my salad with two different types of salsa and the salad was good! I was happy with that, but the salad alone would have been fine.

Sunday night dinner was not happening. Even with that tiny piece of chicken leg, I was well fed and rested after spending a good Sunday evening on the couch. We thought about eating a little something anyway around 9 p.m. to avoid being famished, so I made appetizers. I brought out the two vegan spreads I bought at the farmer's market: the garlic, orange, and ginger spread and the one made from beets. I was hoping Richard wouldn't notice it was beets again, but he asked and I told him. He sneered all right even though he loved it a few days before.

We had rice crackers with the vegan dips and I also made two crab cakes that were no bigger than the size of a half deck of cards each. I read we should only have meat the size of a deck of cards. Well, we had crab cakes half this size and felt as if we were cheating. The crab cakes were our dinner too. It wasn't a lot, but with the white wine we were fine. We're not doing well on this new lifestyle. We're cheating all the time. Something tells me we're at least reducing the amount of food we're eating, but if we're supposed to strive to have plant-based foods, I need to educate myself more.

The next morning, I was reminded that the simplicity of trying to live a healthier lifestyle was a different story.

Chapter 13

Owning Up to It

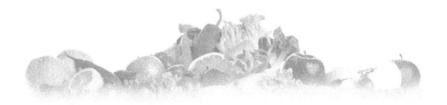

Here we are again and I don't have anything I need to make for breakfast. I'll research this later, I tell myself. For now, I decided to make a shake. How often do we do this? We know what we have to do but put it off. I'm married, but I can't imagine what it would be like with a bigger family or kids with different personalities and tastes. This is a process and I would imagine the more people in the family, the longer the process. We can't go from one extreme to another overnight. According to *Forks Over Knives*, though, some unfortunate but grateful people had to do it to save their lives. The good news is that we can all take small steps. Even if we avoid meat and dairy in our snacking it would be a start.

I added peaches, shake mix, ground flax seed, orange juice, strawberry flavoring, and carrot juice in the mixer. I thought an orange, peach, and strawberry shake would be good, but I think I was found out. Richard didn't like it. Maybe he saw the opened carrot juice? He is pretty picky. On a scale of one to ten, with ten being the pickiest, he would be a seven. Not everyone is going to be so inclined to make the change from strawberries to beets, but slowly, the more we eat healthier, the more I notice we're trying the foods that are good for us. I've always liked the difficult foods—from grapefruit juice, beets, tomato juice, jicama, spaghetti squash, and many other foods a lot of people don't like.

As I've grown older, I've come to like goat cheese, oysters, lamb, caviar, and raw fish. These are not items many people like, but they are an acquired taste. That's the key—acquired. The definition of acquire is: 1. to come into possession or ownership of; get as one's own as to *acquire property*. 2. to gain for oneself through one's actions or efforts: *to acquire learning*. 3. *linguistics;* to achieve native like command of (a language or a linguistic rule or element). 4. *military;* to locate and track (a moving target) with a detector, as radar. If we are to acquire this lifestyle, it looks as if we're going to have to own up to it and acquire the tastes.

It sometimes takes fifteen tries to like these foods, according to the documentary *Vegucated.* In this film, the dietician explains that it can take up to 15 tries to like a certain food. That's how we acquire our tastes to it. I've had to try certain foods in different ways, but the key is trying them again and again. The way I grew to like lamb was how I realized I liked it cooked a certain way. The first time, I wasn't too crazy about it. Lamb is sometimes gamier in some dishes over others. Learning this about lamb, however, I know now to apply this same reasoning with plant-based foods.

For lunch, I reached for the pack of mini baguettes and sliced one in half. The baguette was the cheat with avocado on top. I realized avocado was going to be the sticky staple spread. I added tomato, onion slices, and oregano on top. It was delicious!

I was on my own for dinner so I had free rein to do as I pleased. Richard wouldn't be home for dinner tonight. I realized I didn't have to consider if it was going to be Italian, American, or Mexican. I just thought about what I would eat. I grilled the leftover spaghetti squash that was in the fridge. I sautéed onions and tomato and added seasoning to the spaghetti squash and put that in there too. Done. With some avocado on top, it was not only flavorful, but also colorful and beautiful. I finally began to comprehend what was going on. Was I learning how to eat a plant-based meal yet?

Chapter 14

It's Happening

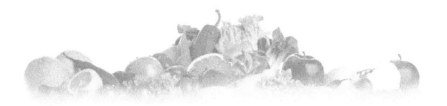

Today I had another epiphany. This morning I made pancakes and offered them to Richard with a pear. I admit that wasn't the best match—pancakes and a pear—but it was the only fruit we had. I realized then we were short on fruits and veggies. I had wondered when I'd gone to the market the last time. Either way, I realized I needed to make sure I stocked up on produce. I would typically buy maybe two bell peppers, salad, four tomatoes, a cucumber, and so on. Now I'm doubling the amount of vegetables I buy as we're going through them quickly. I now buy two to three types of salad, at least two cucumbers, six to ten tomatoes, at least three bell peppers, and a lot more carrots.

I made my pancakes and had my espresso. I didn't mess around with the frother today. I tried to be minimal on the creamer and the thought of adding a drizzle this time in my espresso suited me fine—in my tiny cup that I never use, of course. I have decided to enjoy drinking my morning coffee out of a cup

I like and find my enjoyment that way instead of having several cups with sugar and cream in a mug I can toss. How often do I do this? Does it work? I'll keep applying this theory and see how it pans out.

Lunch was successful! At least that's what I thought. After digging through my fridge, I found a tiny amount of enchiladas. It totaled about one, maybe two, tortillas in a small bowl and with a side of sautéed spinach and garlic it was perfect! I realized I had to skip the cheese melted on top but remembered we still had a lot of Mexican Cotija cheese. I sprinkled a tiny amount over my enchiladas and it was beautiful! It was just the right amount. I would not have hesitated to smother it with cheddar cheese but decided to sprinkle a very small amount of Cotija cheese on top instead.

For dinner, I wanted to make something special and different and I thought; Mahi Mahi steaks, quinoa, and a kale and cabbage salad are what we would have. I tried to create a sweet sauce, but maybe because I was on the phone it didn't come out right. I thought I forgot to add the honey in the marinade of orange juice, pineapple butter, Sriacha, tamari, and fish sauce, but it was the teriyaki sauce that was missing. I may have been distracted, but after doing it again and again I'll know this sauce—not just for fish but also for vegetables and pastas. Nonetheless, we had fish tonight.

If I'm going to learn how to prepare only a plant-based meal someday, I'll have to learn how to make tasty sauces and seasonings, especially if the sauce is a main ingredient to foods. I'm usually good at making sauces, but I was distracted. How many times do we do things right out of habit, though? Was I easily distracted from doing something that needed my attention and focus?

After a while of fixing dishes within our diet choice and sticking as close to the plant-based, whole food diet as we could, it's getting easier if not more familiar to eat this way. It means choosing what is in our fridge and getting more used to the different kinds of foods I've cooked and stored. Instead of choosing between Italian with pasta, pizza, steak, and potatoes, chicken Caesar salad, taco salad, beef tacos, or Mexican, we are choosing spinach, tomatoes, cabbage, kale, beans, quinoa, stir fry, salad, lentil soup, and gluten-free spaghetti with peppers, onions, and garlic sautéed with a natural organic tomato sauce in a jar.

For snacks we have bruschetta, orange, garlic, and ginger vegan spreads, a beet spread, small dishes of chopped beets, rice crackers, and a growing amount of cooked cauliflower, spaghetti squash, spinach, and avocado. Mix all these with a cupboard of not only basic spices but also Chinese Five Spice, Mexican lime chili powder, Chesapeake Bay, Turkish spice, Curry, Cajun spices, and other specialty spices to create a unique flavor.

It doesn't happen overnight, but a new way of eating is happening. For one, I'm learning many more ways to eat a vegetable. I thought adding cheese and tomatoes to all veggies was enough to cook them differently. But apparently it isn't.

Chapter 15

Sweet Potato

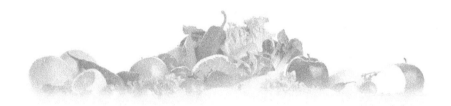

Today was a much better day for sticking to our plan. We still had a bit of a struggle this morning; I'm still having a hard time figuring out what to make for breakfast. We are used to eating eggs almost every day and relished the ham, bacon, or sausage to go with them. You can have only so much fruit when you crave protein first thing in the morning—or at least what we think our only option for protein is.

I stared in the fridge, the freezer, and then the pantry as I normally do. I started to think that whatever healthy sweetness I would find would be great. The mornings usually call for something sweet. The challenge is finding these foods I would normally think to have for lunch or dinner but for breakfast by making them sweet. At least that's what I realized after looking at a list of vegan breakfast items on Google. And, of course, I didn't remember any of them and the thought of finding something I could make sweet caught me in a deep focus.

That's what made me think of a sweet potato. And, yes, I had two! These have been going bad the few times I've bought them because I forget I have them in the corner in a paper bag. So I brought those out and started to think. I took my iPad out and Googled "Yams for breakfast recipes" after putting them in the microwave, peeling them, cutting them into cubes, and partly smashing them. As I began to cut into them, half of them were not soft. I ended up mashing them before noticing that most of the recipes called for cutting them into cubes so I scratched all recipes and thought of mashing them with almond milk like a sweet potato pie. Then I thought, pancakes!

Here's what was interesting. I didn't end up using the almond milk but instead used about a third of what I would normally use of pancake mix with water and half of the potato (who knows how they would turn out with the whole potato?). They came out mushy but good!

I used the ketchup dispenser for the coconut oil that was nice to have on hand and another unique idea for using my binge purchase from the grocery store. It's crazy to think this oil is sold in a jar with a wide cap. It's like buying syrup in a peanut butter jar. (It was warm so the oil melted in the jar like syrup.)

For lunch, I think I had some pistachios, raw almonds that were incredibly sweet, and Naan bread with half bruschetta spread and half vegan beet spread. I probably could have cut up beets and put them on top of the Naan bread, come to think of it, but I'll do that next time.

Dinner was a breeze. It's all about the leftovers now. I had the quinoa from last night. I chopped zucchini, onions, and garlic and sautéed them. At the end, I added tomatoes. For a side dish, I cut a few carrots julienne style and steamed them. I dug through my pantry and thought of adding something sweet. I love to cook. At anytime I can find something I bought long ago and it will be there. I reached way in the back and found a jar of molasses. Every household, whether in a chef's kitchen or a bachelor's, might find a jar of molasses. Does this ever get old? At this point, with what it's made of, probably not. I researched it and must have been reminded. I knew it was raw sugar and what's used to make brown sugar. Why was I still buying brown sugar when I had pounds of white sugar I hadn't used to make my jam preserves? Regardless, I'd have to know if "making" brown sugar is even possible. Is it?

I added about a tablespoon of molasses into the carrots and put the lid on to let them steam. I tossed the day-old quinoa in the pan with the zucchini mix and it looked beautiful. I began to wonder if I should start taking photos and post them. Little did I know why I would later need to see these photos.

Chapter 16

Story of Pain

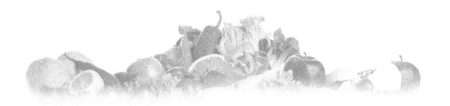

It was a typical morning with coffee, but then I had tea afterward. Not sure what it is, but I do feel more conscientious about what I eat. I'm not sure having tea is the answer to being health conscious, though. My favorite breakfast now is a corn tortilla, avocado, onions, and a little salt. With fruit on the side it becomes a complete breakfast.

It's obvious I haven't been successful at avoiding meat and dairy altogether. But I've been putting a lot of effort into diminishing the amount I use overall and that's been eye-opening. I can't imagine what it's like for those patients who are told to avoid it completely overnight just to live. This is not what I'm trying to do here, for which I'm grateful, but I think over time my use of meat and dairy, mainly meat, will decrease by about 99.9 percent of the time. Not because of the treatment of animals, not necessarily to be more health conscious, nor because I don't like meat or dairy—because I do. I'm not eating meat because we are not meant to eat it every day, the way we're not designed to drink alcohol and eat high-calorie desserts every day. We are not made to have a chocolate ice cream sundae for breakfast, lunch, and dinner.

If I'm in Tuscany or Germany for Oktoberfest, I might be more inclined to be 95 percent meatless instead of 99 percent, the same way I would have a bit of that chocolate sundae at a birthday party. But when I'm eating more than 50 percent meat and calling it a great way to diet I wonder if I'm misinformed. I have to ask, if we weren't in such a capitalistic society (for which, by the way, I'm eternally grateful), would we need to be so dependent on the foods that have historically been a delicacy? This is what goes on in my head as I ponder why I've chosen this way of eating. Choice meats, milk, and cheeses were never for the most poor, were they? Now hundreds if not thousands of years later, with technology and a growing knowledge of how to produce food methodically, have we become a culture where the wealthy, the poorest, and everyone in between are dependent on meat and cheese? I have to wonder if we are coping by simply widening our doorways and chairs. I found a book called *The Cambridge World History of Food,* in a two-volume set and ordered it. The more I understand, the less likely I am to be tempted.

Today was the day to shop for groceries. But as I enter the store, I am no longer walking in the way I used to walk. It may not have been the right advice to shop only on the outer aisles for the foods we're supposed to eat—not when I'm trying to avoid meat and dairy. I would have to pass processed butter, cheeses, packaged foods, the butcher, packaged meats, processed meats, eggs, juices (with more than 23 grams of sugar in each serving), yogurts, sour creams, and even processed, ready-to-bake breads. The bread is typically in the center aisle and that hasn't been good for me either.

Arthritis runs in my family, due to inflamed joints. The worst food I can eat is red meat. The meat is what produces the acid that causes the cartilage in my joints to deteriorate faster from what I understand. I learned from the Celiac Foundation support group that wheat has yeast and genetically modified grains. Wheat is what causes the inflammation of my joints when they rub together. From what I've been told, when the acid from the meat breaks down the cartilage and my joints are inflamed from eating gluten, I can feel a little pain in my joints, enough to irritate me but nothing alarming. This is what I am led to believe causes the pain. I suppose this is when a doctor would prescribe drugs for me, but that's a different book. I'm not at a point where it's that severe, but I get a hint when the back of my neck is sore and stiff and my thumb and pinky get cramped. This may not be the correct evaluation, but it's what makes sense to me from what I've been advised. It's what my grandmother suffered from for years, yet she may never have known the exact foods causing her pain.

So I stroll through the grocery store with all this information running through my head. From my seeing a chiropractor, an acupuncturist, and my general practitioner and learning from a Celiac support group, all the information becomes like a puzzle creating a picture. I then realize the outer aisles are not necessarily the best way to shop anymore. As a matter of fact, none of what I'm used to eating is good for me anymore. At least this is what I'm learning.

Chapter 17

It Was the Car Show

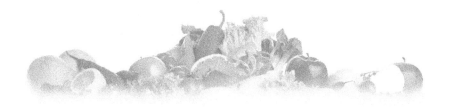

We were both up and going early. I barely had time to drink what has now become my small cup of double-shot espresso and a tablespoon of creamer. It's not nondairy or that chemical creamer either. It's just the organic creamer from Whole Foods I just can't seem to get rid of. A tablespoon is the actual serving size so at least I know I can count my calories if I want to. But I am not interested in counting my calories right now. There's only so much criterion I can take.

We had no time to eat. I grabbed some delicious raw almonds. They're very flavorful and sweet. I added pistachios, water, and a pear to my purse. I have now become a squirrel.

I'm keeping up with our plan to attend a car show at the convention center, but we couldn't get in. We were so frustrated. We drove around and ended up waiting more than twenty minutes in our car only to find out we were in the wrong parking lot. Driving around this convention center, Richard kept grunting that it was all a hoax and a scam and there was no car show; that's how upset he got. After we were told to park miles away at the stadium to be bussed in, we decided to drive back home—a good thirty miles. Then we tried an entrance with no signs—and we got in! We met our brother-in-law and friend of the family and that was when, not surprisingly, we both fell off the wagon.

I'm not sure how alcohol is part of this whole new diet, but I was obliged to accept a drink my brother-in-law offered. Case closed. I'll take the Margarita, thank you. I turned around and there stood Richard with a bag of Oreo cookies and plain potato chips. Really? I suppose the chicken was a gateway for everything available, so why not some junk food snacks? As I'm writing this, I realize it was the frustration that drove us to complete junk food madness.

Dinner was good. We had Chinese food. I did go for pieces of the orange chicken and loaded up on the broccoli. A friend who was there hadn't seen the broccoli and asked where I got it. I know. It's hard to see the green among the orange. We had a lot of dishes laid out in a Chinese buffet style. As much as I stuck with the broccoli and peanuts in the Kung Pow, I still tried the shrimp, chicken, and pork. It was okay. The white wine surely wasn't bad either. It was the weekend and we were with family.

Chapter 18

Crumbs in My Cabinet

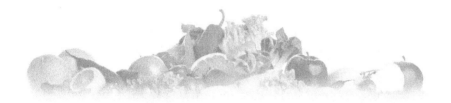

Back at home the next morning, breakfast consisted of half a good shake, but unfortunately I didn't have time to finish it. I tossed spinach, raspberries, chia seeds and shake mix—the usual. It was enough to last until lunch.

As we headed out the door in the late afternoon for a show, we ate the chicken sautéed in onions, bell peppers, and garlic before we left. We're getting used to eating right before we walk out the door, especially if we'll be in a place that has food. I tried to make more vegetables than chicken and I think it came out half-and-half. And that was it. Before, I would always have at least more meat than vegetables, but my mindset is different now. That was the end of the chicken and any other meat except maybe the fish in the freezer I had surprised Richard with already. It was quite satisfying for a Saturday night.

And, yes, we may not be eating completely plant-based, but we're working through this slowly. And who knows? Maybe we'll be eating 100 percent plant-based the more we get used to it. I'm being as optimistic as I can. Having a little fish and sprinkled cheese here and there is like base camp. It's a refuge to what we're used to eating, other than going cold turkey (no pun intended). The chicken we cheated on is how we sigh with a sense of relief between meals. But I'm beginning to think it's more because of the way we are not educated on what to eat or how to eat. We eat chicken because we can't figure out what else to eat. Before we head toward a week of trying to eat primarily plant-based foods, it's as if I were scrounging around before the dead of winter when all I have are crumbs in my cabinet.

We came home at 9 p.m. and were of course hungry. It was late, but we wanted a snack. I thought cherries suggested weeks ago would be great, but I know we wanted something more. I made quesadillas with tomato and spinach and that was enough—almost. To top it off, I made chocolate martinis and that was the end of that. It's amazing how giving in leads to even more disappointment.

Chapter 19

The Upset

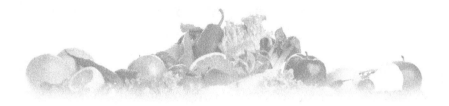

Today was insightful, perhaps because we stuck with the plan. It's the beginning of the week and, I guess, easier to reset. Espresso in the morning was all I had. Richard left in a hurry and didn't even take a banana with him.

When he came home for lunch, though, he was famished and so was I. He grabbed the bread and strawberry jam, but I stopped him. Seriously? I told him I would make lunch. I had no idea what that lunch was, but continuing to eat sugar when nothing else was available was not an option. I was thankful he went on an errand and I started thinking fast. We can't just make sandwiches made of cucumbers. That idea is not something we can venture into quite yet. I know I can't.

I learned today there's a difference between vegan and a plant-based diet. A plant-based diet does not include any processed foods. A lot of vegan foods are processed. Tofurkey, veggie dogs, veggie burgers, and anything that doesn't have meat are processed. I've thought of the veggie sliced cold cuts but for some reason I haven't wanted to try them. And, luckily for me, it's not even considered a plant-based food.

Neither vegan nor plant-based diets include dairy, so processed foods would be the main difference between the two, from what I gather. I see some mention online of food that is "clean," but I'll have to look that up too. That diet name for some reason irritates me. To hear people call this type of diet "clean" is like telling everyone else that what they eat is dirty. Give me a break! I know why I don't follow that "movement." Give it to me straight. Saying you eat clean is retarded.

With that, I've been doing more research, trying to find more recipes, and the photos on Pinterest and Instagram are deliciously attractive. Hands down, vegetarian meals are the most popular on Pinterest. I'm also finding more documentaries. I looked up *Forks Over Knives* and noticed their website and their subscriber e-mail list to get recipes and followed all their social media sites. I looked up documentaries too and added them to my queue on our Netflix account to watch later.

And like the cheeses that were grandfathered into our fridge along with the meats we are working on finishing, I sautéed the processed, disqualifying Mexican style meatless crumble. I think I can make this from scratch. It contains molasses as a binder—I knew it!

I added onions and tomatoes and ate it with some purple cabbage in a tortilla. I made some guacamole too. I'm not sure if it was the cabbage, but I was afraid Richard wouldn't like it. I then remembered the tostadas and smothered guacamole on them, topped it with the meat crumble, added the purple cabbage, and sprinkled some Cotija cheese on top. He loved it. This would be considered a vegetarian dish—we're getting there.

I remembered to soak the red beans and, after they were soaked, I realized they were the same as pinto beans. I still cooked them, but the idea of red beans and rice didn't sound appealing since it was more like pinto beans and rice. In the past, I would have put the whole bag of beans in a Crock-Pot too, but using half the bag was more of what I've learned to do from trial and error.

We had bean burritos with spinach and sautéed onions and peppers. It's been my favorite for a long time. Richard made a face when I added the spinach, but he ate it. He balks at anything green besides broccoli, the only qualifying green he likes.

I shouldn't have had the flour tortillas because my neck stiffens with gluten and it's automatic with flour tortillas in particular. With salsa and a little bit of Cotija cheese we're still working on getting rid of, it was delicious! The cheese in our fridge never ends!

After dinner, I remembered to watch one of the movies again in my Netflix queue. I chose to watch *Vegucated* again. Watching documentaries and educating myself with recipes is opening a whole different way of eating, thinking, and living. I'm almost sure of it.

Watching a simple documentary on the inhumane treatment of animals, as we all know, is heartbreaking. As one of the guys in *Vegucated* said, "You almost have to be completely desensitized" to the way the animals were being treated. Either that or understand you are ignorant. Again, it's all information we commonly know. But like everything else, once we intuitively look into it and think about it, it's a simple decision not to eat meat anymore. I'm processing many reasons, however, other than the awful way these animals are treated and what they have to endure to feed us their bodies. There's a part in this movie where you are taken into the slaughterhouses. The calves are put into these machines and are skinned alive which I wasn't sure why they did that. They are neutered with no pain meds, stuff like that. I still think of these images like the chickens that are clipped into this contraption as they hung upside down. We all know the images. We've seen them.

Second, the intent of this documentary is not just to educate us on the ill treatment these animals go through, but the countless ways that eating meat is doing more harm to our environment. Our generation is so motivated to buy electric cars when not eating meat for a year would yield far more returns to the earth than buying an electric car. Wow. Take that, Prius!

The documentary was so heavy that afterward we decided to watch HGTV to see remodels of homes. We wanted to fulfill our wants rather than our needs. We wanted to watch something comforting to soothe the upset.

Chapter 20

Reheating

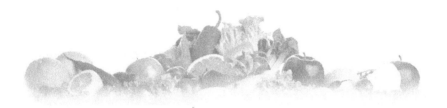

I have to admit I took over this morning. I wanted to use the rest of the sweet potato. I put half in a shake, but it didn't go over too well. It was too thick. I might have to consider pairing it with something less dense than a banana and coconut milk next time.

Regardless, I'm saving more leftovers when I can. We never ate them because after reheating our food it didn't taste the same. Sure, some dishes taste better a day later, like chili rellenos, chili, enchiladas, pizza, stew, but we end up tossing out most of the dishes we save in the fridge.

Although I prided myself on making smaller portions, now I'm saving the bases of food I cook with. Whether it's cooked yams, quinoa, beans, spaghetti squash, avocado, chopped vegetables—eating this way might be simplifying my life. Just maybe. It's completely opposite of what most people think about eating like this. It's actually more time saving that I thought.

I forgot I made coffee. I was too busy concentrating on adding the other half of the yams in the pancake mix. I tried using the electric mixer to see if it would not get too lumpy. It worked fine this time. Regardless, Richard liked them. I had mine later during snack time, but I sprayed I Can't Believe It's Not Butter on my pancakes right out of the pan so I didn't need to add more when I later took them out of the fridge; they were already moist just like I like them. I love butter on my pancakes. Pancakes are not the same without butter. I would have added more butter right after I reheated them, but I didn't this time. Most of the time I'd use stick butter too.

What is interesting is that when I reheated them, I hadn't realized I already sprayed butter on them even though I skipped the butter and just added the syrup. They were delicious. They were moist which is when I realized they already had butter. I ate them with the coffee I had forgotten on the counter, which I didn't finish either. A few swigs of my coffee with pancakes was more than enough.

I need to make something more than just pancakes. I remembered having eggs and polenta so I added polenta on the board hanging on the cupboard. I have a small white board on my cupboard to write down what I'll need from the grocery store. I used to add staples I would run out of, like eggs, meat, cheeses, and yogurts. Now I'm just adding grocery items I need to remember to expand my menus! We're so used to eating meals we've had for years. I now have to recreate our menus. I'd like to experiment more with polenta, chickpeas, and herbs.

For dinner I made pasta with asparagus and mushrooms. The excitement for the day was adding to the asparagus the vegan orange, ginger, and garlic spread I picked up at the farmer's market. I added that as the sauce. Man! It was delicious right out of the pan. I called Richard to tell him how tasty it was, that it was a perfect combination of ginger and garlic added to the mushrooms and asparagus. From the car, he said we probably needed to take out a bottle of wine.

He was stuck in traffic, though. I turned off the stove and waited for him to come home. When he got home, I poured the asparagus mix over the pasta, covered it, and put the dish in the microwave. I had planned to serve it more like a salad mix, but out of habit I forgot and served it like meat sauce.

Unfortunately, this habit didn't serve us well (no pun intended). After heating it in the microwave, it wasn't the same. It came out a little dry and the flavors weren't as good. The wine was too young also, so that didn't suffice either, but of course the bread I toasted was good. I set aside the bread with fresh chopped cucumbers and roasted peppers from a jar.

Some plates are better right out of the pan, not heated up.

Chapter 21

Giving

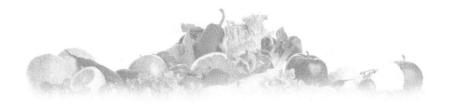

I f I'm the one spearheading this, I should be the only one in the kitchen. If not, I have to prepare myself to be ridiculed for what is or is not in the fridge. If I allow Richard to roam the kitchen, he might say the fridge has nothing in it to eat, the pantry has no chips or cookies, nor does the freezer have any ice cream for that late-night snack. We are only two, but I can't imagine more of us. What I hear most is that we don't have the right sugar drinks or any "good" snacks to munch on. So if he's waiting for breakfast because he's trying to figure it out, I'd better beat him there. These are my first thoughts in the morning.

I reheated the beans and instead of serving them on tostadas, which we had a whole tub of in the fridge, I spread the beans on toast. I didn't think the saltiness of the tostada would work in the morning. I should keep it very light or at least sweet in the mornings from what I remember. Richard doesn't like anything out of the ordinary, especially for breakfast. I could put the refried beans in a flour tortilla, but that would just be another bean burrito. I mashed the avocado into a guacamole and sliced a small portion of onions then layered the guacamole on the beans, adding onions and sprinkling the zesty chili lemon-lime spice on top. I handed it to Richard without making a big deal.

He asked, "beans on toast?" I told him that was how they do it in England, so he took it.

I cut honeydew melon and pineapple and added raspberries in a big bowl for both of us. He asked if the entire bowl was his. (He's kidding, right?) Well, without hesitation, I handed him the entire bowl.

He washed his plate and said it was terrific. While I was making the next beans on toast for myself, I asked if he wanted another one and he asked, "There's more?" Without hesitating, I gave him the one I made for myself.

For dinner, I made a great eggplant Parmesan dish. I love ordering this in restaurants and I've been surprised at how easy it is to cook. I thought I had to soak the sliced eggplant in salt water, coat it with egg and breadcrumbs, and bake it with mozzarella cheese. I always thought there was a long process in making eggplant Parmesan and there probably is. But now I slice the eggplant and throw the slices in the frying pan and they cook just fine, especially with salt, like everything else. It's as if I've been intimidated by this vegetable when it's as easy to cook as zucchini.

I thought about boiling a few tomatoes to make the sauce. This would truly be a whole food, plant-based diet. But my time was limited so, as if I were cheating again, I opened a jar of tomato sauce. Fresh tomato sauce is something I can make on Sunday. I add that to my list of items on the board. The dish was amazing.

This is the whole idea of the WFPB (whole food, plant-based) diet or the PB diet. Avoiding foods with preservatives or foods that are processed is a concept that has been scientifically investigated with significant results. However, Dr. T. Colin Campbell, a leader in these scientific studies, radically claims that his quest of educating the public has been a long and painful road. Anything that is found against government controls will be tested, argued, and shut down. Most of us know this. What many people don't know, though, is that even genetic diseases and some autoimmune diseases can be weakened, including reversing the fate of them.[6]

Adding preservatives is a way for stores to keep things on their shelves for long periods of times as well as in our pantries. I get it. However, we may need more practical ways to cook, because the addition of preservatives to make foods readily available is only beneficial to food companies. Let's be real. With the use of cooking utensils, appliances, and storage ideas such as airtight containers, it's no longer necessary to buy foods with preservatives if I want to take advantage of eating a plant-based diet. If having whole foods without ingredients I can't pronounce would allow the natural process of foods to penetrate my blood stream not so much efficiently but *effectively*[7]—that is what makes sense to me. It's the way I understand good health is supposed to look like, which makes perfect sense to utilize new kitchen gadgets, appliances, and tools available today.

---

6   Dr. T. Campbell wrote in *The China Study*, published by Benbella Books, Inc., a chapter called "Turning off Cancer" 43-67 and later recognizes support: 237 from Hildenbrand GLG, Hildenbrand LC, Bradford K, et al. "Five year survival rates of melanoma patients treated by diet therapy after the manner of Gerson: a retrospective review." *Alternative Therapies in Health and Medicine 1 (1995): 29-37.*

7   In *The China Study*, the scientific definition between "high quality" proteins such as meats is defined as scientifically efficient but often misunderstood by the general public. Plant foods are the better *quality* in terms of having better protein effects. *House of Proteins: 30-31.*

Chapter 22

Grocery Day

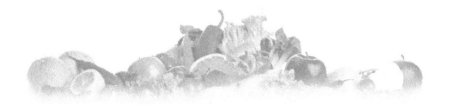

G oing to the grocery store is no longer the big grocery day where I pack a full load of groceries into the shopping cart. The list I create for grocery shopping now has such an array of foods that I may go to the main grocery store for the basics, the specialty health store for the items that are hard to find at a typical grocery store, or even the dollar store to find more expensive items that would be a lot less. And this doesn't have to be done all in one day either. Going to different stores is not any different from what we are used to with the different types of stores that are out there. We have warehouse stores, along with the varied grocery stores we go to for whatever reason, such as health food stores, specialty stores with a cult following, and all kinds of delivery food stores that can deliver anything from diapers to rice.

Before our new way of eating, the grocery list would include eggs, milk, bread, a toiletry, salad, tomatoes, onions, meat, cold cuts, or even just "meat." Now I list items like garbanzo beans, polenta, sesame seed oil, bean sprouts, shallots, coconut water, panko crumbs, sesame seeds, eggplant, tahini, chia seeds, and so many more items than before. I may have some sauces, but most sauces can be made and stored in the fridge and are a lot more economical to make. The difference is adding more foods to what we know, not necessarily taking typical foods off our list, except maybe the more expensive items like meat and cheese. It's hard to understand why people believe that if you avoid meat you have very little to eat when the opposite is true. As I've avoided meat, I've learned of so many more foods and more varied ethnic foods than before.

I'm used to making for example, American, Italian, Mexican, and Chinese. With a change in diet, I'm scrambling to make Thai, Indian, Korean, Vietnamese, Persian, Mediterranean, South American, African, and even, heaven forbid, vegetarian. The world opens up to a whole array of foods to explore but primarily with a plant-based mindset.

Instead of buying three or four tomatoes, I may buy ten. Tomatoes can be boiled and mixed in the blender for fresh tomato sauce from what I've discovered (I just mentioned this a few pages ago). Not a lot of people have time, but I will try this on a weekend and store it in the fridge.

Today, I did buy a roasted chicken. Richard was really hungry and I thought the chicken would be a treat. He's not only been supportive but is also convinced with the information he's been learning. What's crazy is what we classify as a treat these days, but this is the shift in our mindset. We have gone from having chicken a few times a week to maybe only once to once every two or three weeks if at all. I think the more we change our eating habits, the more we will have very little chicken if at all anymore. A lot of people have lived without it for years, if not their whole lives. And I'm sure we would survive fine without it, if not better.

We had a chopped salad with chicken over tostadas and we relished it. You'd think we were indulging on a rack of lamb, but I guess our way of indulging is changing too.

Chapter 23

I Am What I Eat

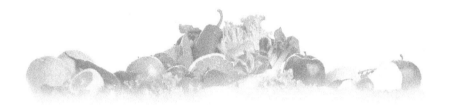

Saturday morning I had a shake. A friend of mine was telling me about her shake as all my friends do. I guess we're in that mid-forties age range when it's the thing to do. Either that or it's "all the rave" with the various shake mixers out right now. Every kind of shake mixer in every color is available. Mine is red. It looks nice, but it scares me sometimes. The first time I turned it on, the bottom part went flying off because the nuts weren't screwed in right after I took it out of the box. I guess it's a sign of how fast they are being made these days.

I usually put spinach in my shakes. From what some folks have said, if you add spinach this makes you "hard core." Well, if you eat sausages wrapped in bacon or have bacon in a hamburger, that should make you hard-core too, right? Like everything else, it depends on what side of the spectrum of hard core you are or whom you hang out with and if it even means something positive.

The shake had spinach, cucumber, apples, chia seeds, coconut water, and lemon. I later texted my friend and told her I tried her shake recipe. She reminded me to add lime because the lime made it more refreshing. I hadn't thought to add lime instead of milk or shake mix. Many of my ideas I get from talking about the change in our diet are with friends. They may add new ideas and twists. When I talk of "diet," it's not temporary. Diet has a number of different definitions, but I choose the definition that describes the habitual partaking of healthy eating as do my friends. You are whom you hang out with.

If I didn't have anyone to get advice from or swap recipes with, it would be hard to be stimulated to find new ideas. The good news is that I have found Google to be the ultimate resource for ideas and recipes and possibly the best partner in this endeavor.

The afternoon was filled with a lot of errands and, of course, dinner was right after. We did the Costco run and went to pick up polska kielbasa for a harvest festival where we were asked to bring European food and because Richard's ancestry is German, sausages were on the menu. It was our attempt at finding something similar to the German wurst. We stopped later at a German deli where they had some fantastic deli meat and sausages and we found a great bratwurst. Since they served lunch and dinner also, we decided to have dinner there too.

I decided to stick to my guns and refused to eat any meat even though we were there picking up sausages. Richard, on the other hand, went for it. How can I give him a hard time when he's connecting to his roots? I ordered the Muenster and tomato grilled sandwich. It was delicious with butter on grilled bread. I had it with a side of fruit.

With that, of course, I felt very full and tired and wanted to fall asleep. I'm allergic to gluten and knew I was overdoing it. I remembered what I was told in the Celiac Foundation support group I was a part of (I don't have Celiac, but I learned a lot about gluten allergies). The more I eat gluten, the more it may be what's causing my neck to stiffen and the more damage it may cause. What that damage is or what more it will cause, I have yet to know. All I know is that my neck stiffens so much that I can hardly turn my head, so I avoid bread 95 percent of the time when I really should avoid it altogether.

Chapter 24

Harvest

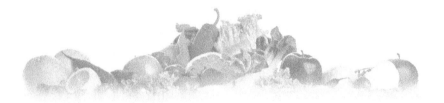

S unday was church day and our annual harvest festival. Here we go! The one thing I'm learning about sticking to a regimen is the amount of effort it takes. There's no room for being lazy, or a losing mentality will seep in and who wants that? Who wants to be asked how one's diet is going, only to respond with, "Yeah, I decided I was going to stick with my original eating habits because it was too hard."

With that, I attempted to make French toast that was dairy-free and gluten-free in the morning while grilling the sausages for the annual harvest festival. Although it sounds a bit extreme, the gluten-free, dairy-free French toast worked. I Googled the recipe and went for it. I used the gluten-free bread I bought at Costco and mixed coconut milk, ground flax, xanthan gum, vanilla, and cinnamon. I added a little bit of the vanilla dietary shake mix for good measure. I dipped the bread and let it cook. For some reason it took longer than normal to cook. Maybe it's the absence of egg that doesn't burn as fast as I thought.[8]

We had them with syrup and raspberries and I posted it on Pinterest and Facebook. Richard and I both liked it.

I knew I would be tempted to eat the bratwurst, polska kielbasa, and pork and veal sausages. I had prepared them in aluminum pans in a chafing wire rack with candles underneath to serve them warm. Not only that, but I had to grill them ahead of time while cooking the French toast. The polska kielbasa, which isn't even German, turned a nice brown-red color and looked delicious! Who am I kidding?

We went to the harvest festival and our sausages didn't last. They were the first to go before the pasta, the salad, the breads, and even the desserts. One teen had two sausages on her plate and that's all. No mustard needed.

I piled on the salads, the German (rotkohl) red cabbage I'd made, and the potato salad and had the smallest white bratwurst. It was the saltiest, most delicious part of my plate, probably because of its saltiness. The meat is the salt. It's no wonder since, according to Wikipedia, 77 percent of the sodium eaten is in processed foods and restaurant foods, 11 percent from adding it to foods or when we cook, and the rest found naturally in other foods. But using information on Wikipedia has to be taken with a grain of salt (no pun intended). Someone told me I couldn't take anything from that site seriously sometimes. (What next?)

Lately, I've been using a lot more salt when I cook. In the past, I didn't need to use so much salt, but I've noticed now that cheese and meat add saltiness to my food—the crumbled Cotija cheese, for sure. Perhaps those on low-sodium diets should avoid cheese altogether because the added salt is an important additive that avoids the growth of bacteria when cheese is produced. And you think the Europeans aren't on this? There was a study published in the British Medical Journal (The *BMJ*) that found the "salt content in cheese sold throughout the

---

8 The recipe for gluten-free and dairy-free French toast is at the back of the book under "Breakfast."

UK was remarkably high despite these products meeting government goals on salt reduction."[9]

The day didn't stop there. Dinner was later with the family at our favorite Italian restaurant that has the best pepperoni bread appetizer there is. Since I primarily had salads for lunch, I was pretty hungry too. The pepperoni bread is basically dough baked with pepperoni and served with either meat or marinara sauce for dipping. We were celebrating a birthday, so to join in the festivities, I had the pepperoni bread with marinara sauce. Richard was surprised I ordered only an appetizer and bread, but the pepperoni bread was enough. I ordered a side of steamed vegetables and my sister was already on my case. She said, "You're not ordering vegetables are you?" She was surprised that I would be ordering vegetables at our favorite Italian restaurant known for their pepperoni bread, pizza, and pastas. I offered her some and she took half.

I could talk about how great the pepperoni bread was, but I don't think I remember eating it. Even though I wouldn't want to remember what pepperoni is made of and that it's one of the worst meats to eat as far as sausages are concerned, it seemed like I inhaled it anyway. I was devouring it at such a rapid pace. I was like a starving lion finally finding its fawn to devour.

Chocolate cake and red wine were also enjoyed and I relished all of it for the night, as did Richard. Instead of ordering the usual spaghetti and meatballs for himself, he surprisingly ordered the shrimp fettuccini. Maybe he thought the seafood was better than the meatballs he'd normally order with spaghetti but regardless, it was a change and I took notice.

---

9   It's not that difficult to find research on cheese and salt. This study was founded by one of the leading British medical journals online at www.bmjopen.bmj.com under the Archive tab, Vol 4, Issue 8 article on Cross-sectional survey of salt content in cheese: a major contributor to salt intake in the UK.

Chapter 25

Just Know This

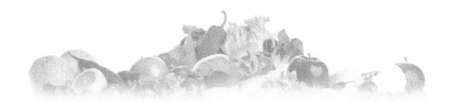

As I close out the month, the number of challenges that led to insights and beliefs was astounding. After starting this, I thought I would learn a few things, but I didn't realize how many discoveries I would make. If I could list them all, would it help change the way people eat? Would it help people understand the importance of writing down everything, no matter what?

We need cooking utensils, appliances, and gadgets that can help us dice, chop, and mince because we don't know how. Companies are getting rich because they're depending on us not to know how to cook or what to spend on kitchen utensils. I like to think I know how to cook even though I love kitchen gadgets but if you don't know how to cook, at least you know there are cooking gadgets for you on just about anything you need help with.

We are not 100 percent plant-based, vegetarian, or even gluten-free. Richard and I are rather more educated and a tad healthier and we have more options from consciously *trying* to eat plant-based. We now actually respect those who strictly follow this type of diet and hold no stereotypes or prejudices against them. We get it.

I no longer buy meat or eggs and when I do, they sit in my fridge for weeks. When my husband buys a good sandwich, he brings the other half home to me. Truth is, I think we're just getting used to eating without meat and dairy.

I would recommend trying to adhere to a plant-based diet for a month to learn how to eat healthy. Trying this diet for a month has stretched my knowledge of plant-based foods and recipes. Our palate has changed and so have our habits. What we once thought incapable is now welcomed, such as cucumbers in a vegetarian sandwich. I suppose our bodies have adapted to it. And when I put mind over matter I started to put mind over food. We were stretched. We failed. We argued and then we complained. Now my husband questions me as to why I revert to eating the way we used to if I decide to cheat like I normally do. My husband who was my initial complainer is now the plant base police if I stray from what I'm advocating because I get tired and feel the need to have a piece of chicken or cheese.

My husband is not a natural at this and neither am I. But we want to be healthy. We don't want the burden of illnesses if we can help it. If we are fortunate to be in a generation that can spread the word, save our planet, reduce medical insurance costs, and save lives, then this is the reason for this book.

I wanted to understand a way to eat healthier and to incorporate a different lifestyle. I wanted to understand how people were able to eat the right foods all the time as if it were a habit. I wanted to sit in a lab to learn how I would react, what choices I'd make, and tie them into the physics and chemistry of the foods so this knowledge would be ingrained in my psyche. Do you know these people? How do they do it? That's what I wanted to find out. Were they this disciplined, or is there something more behind the psychology of what they believed?

The only way to change our eating habits is to change our minds. But the only way to change our minds is to change our behavior. We won't register a good diet until we experience, stretch our knowledge, and, as they say, struggle the way a butterfly does to live. You go to college for the experience, not necessarily for the degree, right?

We will have to close our eyes to the abundance, take a stand, be disciplined, and make that choice to try as hard as we can to understand what a plant-based diet is. I hope I have given you insight because, looking back, I don't know what all the negative hype was about. Eating your vegetables is not a big deal, but people make it a big deal. When we have steak, pasta, and eggs, who's arguing about that? Not many people are.

It was trying something so simple I thought was so hard, like a child not wanting to eat their vegetables. It's not the vegetable itself but how it's cooked. I learned how to like them more and to choose them over meat. I once heard a top chef say steak was boring because all you can do is chew on it. I thought at the time it was interesting for him to say that. Now I know. You have so much more to experience and savor out there that, once you know, you rarely go back. It's like traveling for the first time after years of never going and, now that you've been overseas, you're hooked!

How else are we supposed to like our vegetables? As we grow older, aren't we supposed to learn how simple eating our vegetables is? Let me explain. Will we no longer make a funny face when we have roasted carrots as a main entrée or wonder what it's like not to have meat or dairy for dinner? Will we no longer question eating vegetables all the time? We will only know by getting used to it and go about our daily lives without much thought about living a plant-based diet. That's how.

It's good to write down everything you eat every day, but it's more effective when you journal about it. How do you feel? What do you question? What have you researched? It's like data that does not lie. The truth to your not being able to change your diet is in the raw data. It's your beliefs about meat and dairy, like your salvation. What you discover and what you articulate when you read what you ate will change how you eat. Your body will tell you more, though.

If you're having problems losing weight, cut the meat and dairy for a month. Call it the "I'm-Getting-Educated-on-How-to-Eat Diet." If you discover how tragic it is that you don't know what else to eat, then you'll know why you have a hard time losing weight and staying healthy. The answers to your problems will be in the data—in your journal.

And last, but certainly not least, are the many varieties of white fish that are supposed to be, another great metabolism-boosting source of protein; the latest information I am learning from the experts. I've always understood fish to be a major player when it came to eating healthier, but high levels of contamination and mercury found in fish can cause a lot of damage and can be toxic.

Although mercury acts slowly, it builds up over time, typically in the heart. Although fish has been promoted as being necessary for heart health, it's actually been found to be the opposite. "In one study, mercury levels were 15 percent higher among those patients who had suffered a first heart attack. A second study showed increased risk of cardiovascular mortality with increasing mercury exposure. The third study found that a high content of mercury in hair might be a risk factor for acute coronary events, cardiovascular disease, coronary heart disease, and all-cause mortality in middle-aged men. This study also found that mercury may negate the purported protective effects of fish on heart health."[10]

This diet, way of eating, experiment or whatever you want to call it should not be construed as my belief in "the only way" to eat. As I mentioned, it has only been proven to dramatically decrease or heal illnesses. However you want to look at it, whether myth, an opportunity, or complete lie, we cannot deny that if we learn how to eat vegetarian or a whole food, plant-based diet, we will be better off. My point is that by trying, I've discovered how uneducated I was in trying to incorporate more plants and vegetables in my diet although it's been perfectly "normal" with how I eat with others. I thought, "How hard can this be, to eat a diet of vegetables, grains, and fruits?" It was hard! So from this exercise, I learned there's no denying we need to prioritize cooking as we do our finances or

---

10 All these studies were written in an article found from Physicians Committee for Responsible Medicine website: wwwpcrm.org/health/reports/fish. The first study was documented from: Guallar E, Sanz-Gallardo MI, van't Veer P, et al. Heavy Metals and Myocardial Infarction Study Group. Mercury, fish oils, and the risk of myocardial infarction. *N Engl J Med.* 2002; 347: 1747-1754.

The second study was documented from: Salonen JT, Seppanen K, Nyyssonen K, et al. Intake of mercury from fish, lipid peroxidation, and the risk of myocardial infarction and coronary, cardiovascular, and any death in eastern Finnish men. *Circulation.* 1995; 91: 645-655.

The third study was documented from: Virtanen JK, Voutilainen S, Rissanen TH, et al. Mercury, fish oils, and risk of acute coronary events and cardiovascular disease, coronary heart disease, and all-cause mortality in men in eastern Finland. *Arterioscler Thromb Vasc Biol.* 2005; 25(1): 228-233.

plan a vacation if we want to improve our health overall. We can't deny that we need to invest in our health. This means that we need to take a close look at not only how we eat but in learning how to cook, not just by picking up the latest most popular diet because of how someone else did on it.

This book was not intended to convert you completely to a plant-based diet, tell you why it's better to be plant-based, or make you feel any less because you're not converting. My journey shows you how we are trying to eat a plant-based diet and incorporate it into our daily meals and it has shown us how many recipes we didn't know. It got me to stretch myself to learn it. We can learn how to eat better only by understanding, being educated, and seeing how much we don't know. Only through this process were we able to let go of fad diets and truly live a healthier life. Can the answer to losing weight and getting healthy go beyond a popular diet and exercise? I think it can.

It's like this: You have an expensive luxury car. You use leaded gas instead of premium, hardly give it a detail wash, and are constantly overloading and packing it. Every so often, you are inclined to run it fast to remind you how fast it can go but in the end, the car, as beautiful as it is, doesn't look the same or run the same after awhile and you can't go long distances in it anymore. If it's the wear and tear, the misuse and ill-guided information that ruins your car, it is the same in how we take care of our bodies. Does this make sense?

Well, here is my attempt at describing further.

Part II

THE FINDINGS

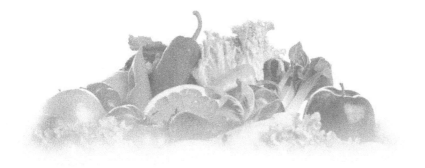

Chapter 26

Failure

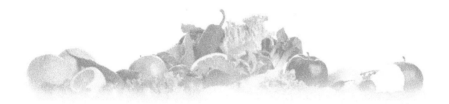

F ailure is not such a bad thing. Throughout the entire month or so, we experienced more failure than I thought we would. The amount of guilt also plays an important role. It's been helpful for me to write and then read about the guilt. It has come in handy when reaching for that cheese at the grocery store or around friends. Guilt has worked like a shock treatment. I've chosen to pay attention to it instead of deny it. It came with the territory.

Unless the doctor orders a change in one's diet, changing the diet will take time. Together, Richard and I both accepted our failures in our eating habits and moved on. We always had the next day. We had an extreme amount of failure, though—a lot more than I had anticipated. The good news is that getting a head start on it now before a doctor decides for us is probably the best choice. Life has no guarantees. If we have to resort to this in the future, we'll be prepared, like preparing for "the big one" here in California. We never know.

For most people, failure becomes the end-all, but it doesn't have to be. I see failure as a way to help us continue on a journey of a healthier diet, so it becomes okay. It was interesting to see how much failure we endured but were still able to change our eating habits, and that is significant. We failed in front of friends and with each other but what consequences did we really suffer? None. Through this process, I was actually able to change because I got so tired of the after effects. Let failure drive you and continue on.

Failure has been the key that keeps us on this journey. Like they say, the only failure is when you stop trying.

Chapter 27
Dishes

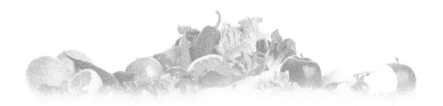

F irst, I'm now enjoying dishes I've always had in my cabinets—from espresso cups I never thought I'd use to the Asian bowls I had on a shelf that looked pretty. When I backed up my belief about knowing I should stop the creamer, the way I stopped using sugar in my coffee, I naturally began to enjoy my espresso cups, including my espresso maker. After all, I'm on my third espresso maker.

The small, pretty Asian bowls are now used for rice or vegetables since they are the right size. The small cups I received as a wedding gift are the perfect size for enjoying a small cup of coffee. These cups were the only set of dishes Richard and I agreed to on our wedding registry too. With all the time we put into deciding which set of dishes to include in our registry, we only made out with two cups in this set that had been stored in the cupboards until now.

What dishes do you have that are in your cabinets that you never use? What did you buy with good intentions but because of your habits, you never use them? I was surprised that I had all the right intentions to use dishes that I kept for the right reasons but because of our lifestyle, I just never enjoyed them.

Or how about the appliance you bought but have never used? Is it a wok, a rice cooker, a steamer that you have all the right intentions of using but never do? Is it still siting in your cupboards?

I found that when I changed my eating habits, I was dusting off these dishes, appliances and tools as a warm welcome to a long lost gem.

Chapter 28

Leftovers

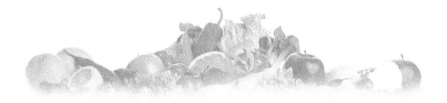

W e almost never ate leftovers. It was rare when we did, but we'd always store them anyway. As they say, it feels better to throw away food-gone-bad. We never even looked for leftovers before they'd go bad. Now I'm not only looking for leftovers, but I'm also looking for something already cooked to add to my dishes. I'll store cooked potatoes, spaghetti squash, sweet potato, cooked quinoa, beans, anything I can add to what I'm cooking. I can add sautéed spinach with leftover enchiladas. Sure, you may already do this, but is it a habit? Or are you like me? Do you find something already spoiled that you could have used had you seen it?

Do you cook only for that one time you are eating or do you cook for the next few days within that hour or so you are cooking? A key habit to healthy eating is actually in the leftovers and the amount you have that is readily available in your fridge. What I have found remarkable is how much I combine different ingredients and foods in one dish. Whether it's a soup, fried rice, a burrito or a casserole, forget the ordinary lettuce salad – everything becomes some sort of a salad.

Chapter 29

Support

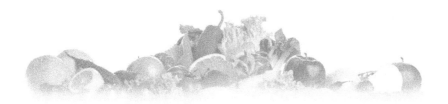

Whether it's family or a roommate, it's essential to find support from those with whom you live. It's important for those around you to support you, but it's crucial for those you live with. Whether it's your family or your roommate, you will forever be climbing an uphill battle if they don't support you and this goes both ways. I found it equally important for me to share the information I'm learning, to be gracious with sharing my food, and to be supportive when they also try but fail.

Will your husband or kids eat their fruit if its cut? Is it better to add BBQ sauce to a veggie dish? This diet doesn't happen overnight but what if we thought of this as a transition, a mere education in food rather than a "strict diet?" My sister is on a Mediterranean diet which is helping her substitute healthy foods over others. I want to tell her it's more simple than that but regardless, I think that's awesome. It's a step in the right direction and it's where she's at. Why would I tell her that she needs to eat plant-based instead? I want to support her endeavors as she supports mine.

If we're going to promote loving our animals, saving the earth and helping humanity, let this drive the cause instead of negating everyone else's choice in how they eat. Sooner or later if this concept becomes more popular which I'm already seeing it is, let the culture win. Not you. You just do what you need to do.

Chapter 30

Groceries

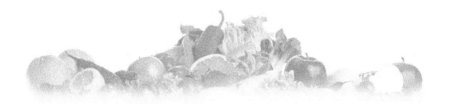

My grocery list was always changing; there were no more of the same items on there again and again. What I decide to pick up at the store grows my knowledge and makes me search for a recipe, like digging for gold. If my list doesn't change, though, it can take me further back from where I started. And when I'm hungry, isn't that the best time to learn? It starts with our grocery list. Whatever I find interesting to eat, I'll add it to my grocery list.

Finding the basic essentials to replace the milk, butter, eggs, meat, cold cuts, and processed foods has been the most challenging. Eggs are used as a binder but are often replaced with natural yeast. I found an egg replacer. That's what it said on the box. I've used xanthan gum too because it's gluten-free. I use avocado instead of sour cream and cheese that glues everything together in tacos. I replace a dairy-based shake mix with water and lime and plant-based milks like coconut, almond, rice, soy, and even grain milk in place of dairy milk. I'm so glad I didn't have to go to the library or the bookstore or get a degree in nutrition. I was making a recipe that called for plant milk and that was foreign to me. I hadn't heard of that before. I had to do an online search by typing, "What is plant milk?" I'm not kidding. I truly had no idea. However, it was that simple to find out, but it taught me how much I'm not used to the basic terminology.

Cheese in the fridge lasted us a whole month before we were totally out of it. Before, it would have been gone in a week because it was normally on our grocery list every week. Now I understand what rationing is. That's what it seemed like with the cheese, though I always felt guilty when we used it during my first month. I hadn't realized how much cheese we had, but after watching a few documentaries I gave it a second thought. Shredded cheese is not good for you if you're gluten-free because some of the machines that grate the cheese are sometimes used for gluten-based foods. That's what I learned from the Celiac Foundation support group. Eliminating cheese altogether is probably the hardest part. Nothing is like it. But, like meat, it has a lot of salt and although salt is necessary, the human body is not prepared to accept so much salt in our diets. Salt goes beyond just adding it at the table. Salt is in meats, cheeses, breads, and pastas and by adding more salt to our foods, we easily over indulge.

My mother-in-law was so opposed to using salt on our foods and she never cooked with it. My husband is good at not overdoing it on salt because he was used to it being the enemy. My mother-in-law swore that salt was bad for you till the day she passed, but like my grandmother, I wonder if she knew more about the foods that were causing her to feel that way. Regardless, she held this conviction close to her heart—perhaps because she lived during the food-rationing era after World War II during Germany's hyperinflation. Milk and dairy were probably not as available and as a child, along with her family; at times she had to rummage through the potato fields for leftovers just to eat. When she probably started having meat and dairy again, especially after coming to the states when she was already nine years old, these foods probably tasted very salty to her. I can certainly relate to that now.

Sprinkling Cotija cheese on our tacos gives it that burst of salt flavor I had never experienced before. When you go without meat or dairy and then have cheese again, it tastes very salty. To this day, if I buy turkey deli meat, I'm more inclined to have it without the salt additives. My taste buds have certainly changed.

Chapter 31

Research

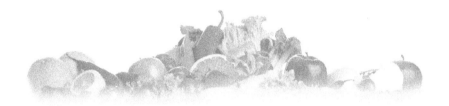

I don't think I could have gone farther down this road had there not been Google. We are now without excuses. If an idea for potato tacos comes to mind, searching for a recipe for potato tacos[11] in Google reveals choices for vegetarian, plant-based, spicy, or breakfast potato tacos. The amount of information is infinite. My iPad or even my iPhone often came to the rescue. Almost all devices have the Internet; in our house with only two people, we always have something to pick up and Google right away in the kitchen.

I'm not a chef, but I'm constantly looking for anything new to try at restaurants for ideas. I want to taste how persimmons are prepared in a salad and how polenta with mushrooms comes out. Sometimes I can get used to ordering the same dishes on a menu because it's what I'm used to; it's all I know and want to know. If we find something that sounds interesting, are we more inclined not to try it because it's just not what we're willing to take a risk on paying for?

---

11   I added the recipe in the last section under Dinner.

I have found that I'm searching for plant-based dishes that I'd like to try to find more ideas on how to cook. I'm like a student, curious to see how something is made to see if I can broaden my menu at home. I'll pick up vegan spreads with different combinations like ginger and orange and try them with different vegetables even if they're a little more expensive although I know I'm still under budget than I used to be. Better yet, I want to replicate this spread and make it myself. I want to make farmers markets more a priority too to learn more what others are making.

Downloading any kind of movie or documentary that will help me understand more about why cheesy, warm, and delicious pizza is not good for us is a quest too, though I'm not sure I would abstain completely from pizza. Going out for pizza on Friday nights is still our treat. However, I'll try a pizza with capers, fresh tomato, and spinach in a restaurant to see if I could add that to my list of things to incorporate in my food at home.

I tried a pineapple, banana, and peanut butter shake in a café and it was absolutely delicious. I was stumped this morning on what to make yet I had all these ingredients to make this delicious shake. The fact I had all these ingredients to make something great and was clueless about what to have for breakfast proves I have so much more to learn.

We need more education, more promotions, more of a movement like establishments such as Whole Foods have done—although they are sometimes scrutinized. Do we think they are the only grocery store that has been caught mispricing their items at the register?

Chapter 32
Kindness and Generosity

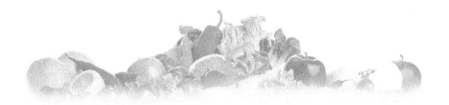

Simple kindness can be the hardest to achieve during this process of transition, although it has been absolutely necessary to see this through. The more kindness, the more accomplishment there is. With generosity, we are able to embrace this new diet—at least just for the two of us. Don't mess with hunger. A hungry appetite between two people can be a terrifying duo. Be generous. If he's liked it, I've given it to him—even if it's my portion. Do whatever it takes. Being nice at least helps me to be more attractive even when I'm around those who rebel against this way of eating. This is an exciting journey if we have fun with it too. I tried as hard as I could to make sure foods tasted good, but if you don't like it, don't serve it.

On the other hand, don't be such a promoter either. Just serve the food. If they ask, tell them to try it first. As smart mothers do for their children, we should do for those we love, no matter how old they are. I wasn't afraid to say, "Try it—you'll probably like it." Or, "Who cares what it is if you like it?" Be brave and bolder, but understand there is a psychology behind why they don't like it too, not only because it doesn't taste good. My husband had three platefuls of tongue I made when we first got married but he said he felt sick to his stomach only after I told him what it was. He hasn't eaten it since, but I can tell you he liked it and devoured it.

When I'm reading what other say about their diets and why they're the best, it's contradictory when they become rude with their rants online. I find this very hypocritical when a big reason to avoid meat is to be kind to animals. We want to love animals and the earth but we can be so rude to each other. Keep in mind that a plant-based diet promotes kindness and generosity but can only confuse those who are trying to hear the message.

Chapter 33

Frying

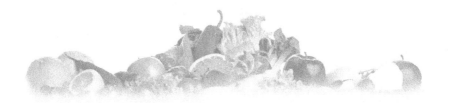

I use only coconut oil when sautéing. Buy it. Buy the unrefined kind too. It is a little expensive and outrageously expensive at Costco because of the quantity you have to buy although I've just recently found this more affordable there for some reason. If I absolutely must sauté my foods for stir-fry, at least I'm using the stuff most recommended. The most up-to-date news is that if we have to cook with oil, it's the only oil that will work in our favor when heated at high temperatures. Again, you can Google this and find out more but as I'm writing this, it's supposed to be the best oil to use for frying. Who knows? Even that can change though.

Coconut oil helps to make the food more flavorful. I got so used to this flavor that any other kind of oil may not only reverse what I'm trying to do with my health, but it won't taste the same. I'm sautéing too, not frying, and have replaced butter with coconut oil on my pancakes. However, after learning that oils don't qualify for a plant-based diet, I will have to be even more creative in my cooking.

Honestly, just by trying, it can help to diminish bad habits. If we can just substitute the oils in the beginning, and just write down what triggers our subconscious by using a different oil, maybe the frying won't be that important anymore. Either it's the cost of the oil or the taste that will affect us. Which is it? These are things to write about in a journal. Would you think differently about frying if it's costing you more because coconut oil is not as cheap as canola oil? Would you fry on the weekends only or maybe once a month because of the cost or, would it not matter at all? Will you still pay the price of expensive coconut oil, the health effects of frying with canola oil or both? Why?

Chapter 34

Wine

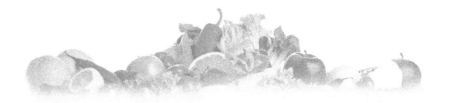

I s wine plant-based? Why, yes and no. I've just recently learned more about how wine is made and what's in it.[12] However, the same rule that is known to all applies: Don't over drink! Richard and I try not to drink too much wine even though we've heard one glass every night is fine. The problem with wine is the same as cheese. If you have too much of it, you'll always want to drink it and your tolerance will only get higher. You know this.

I haven't researched organic wine, but the process of making it is unique to some wineries for this reason. If you were a wine connoisseur, understanding the process of wine making would be part of you being able to hold that title. True wine lovers have a good understanding of wine making and will know if it's truly vegan or not although a lot of times the sommelier or the vendor who you are buying it from will know too. It's certainly a great area for you to research more

---

12   We just learned that animal products such as eggshells are used to filter the wine during the final process. I'm so glad I'm not a strict vegan.

if you don't know enough about it. We enjoy wines and learning about them but I wish I could say the healthier we are in our eating, the more disciplined and watchful we have become with drinking wine, but we are not. We drink wine whether it's been processed with or without animal products.

What I have come to realize from learning about wine however, is that the savviest wine drinkers understand the chemistry behind the flavors of food, in particular, farm to table foods. And a plant-based diet appeals to this audience because of the different tastes one wine bottle can have depending on what is paired with it. There's nothing like a dinner in the vineyard with local farm fresh foods and vegetables that are married with great tasting wine. From salads with radicchio and capers to butternut squash with pecans and coconut oil and brick oven artisan bread, corn on the cob with olive oil and thyme and wild rice with a homemade dressing; the art of food is color, the look, and of course the different mouth-watering tastes. Whether it's meat or produce that is locally grown, this is what puts Northern California on the map and why we eventually bought a home there. People from all over the world come to see what this is all about.

Wine pairing creates wonderful experiences of tastes like a healthy diet of fruits and vegetables when they are either eaten raw or cooked in ways to make the true tastes come out. There really is no need for melted cheese to steal the show unless you're having a sliced piece of cheese made by a local farmer just large enough to wash it down with a pinot noir. On the other hand, a healthy plant-based diet and great wine make for a great marriage whether on the vineyard or in your home.

If you have been lucky enough to experience great wine pairings with remarkable wines with farm to table foods, then you will understand how it's the chemistry that develops in every mouthful and not just the food you eat by itself that enhances your experience. Just like how a steak has to be seasoned, if your plant foods are paired with other plants and grains, the combinations of taste are amazing. There are different tastes that are found in healthy foods that are infinite, and when you wash it down with different wine varietals, you will know.

Chapter 35

In Summary

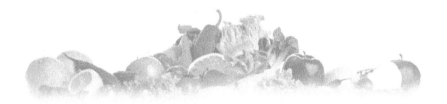

I wish I could say I gave an account on every single day, but for the sake of being too boring, I think I wrote enough after the twenty-sixth day. I wanted to write just enough not to make this too long for the average person who will read this book. The truth is, I tried to add every epiphany, every discovery, and everything important I wanted to express. All things considered, I wrote what I thought needed to be written.

I gave us four weeks to empty the fridge of all dairy and meats, including cheeses and milk, but understand this: Although we believe we don't have to abstain completely, we hardly eat any of it anymore. We just don't need to. We were surprised at how long it took to completely eliminate the cheese and meat before we were finished with it. The guilt of eating any cheese for at least a month worked as a stimulant. However, unless our doctor tells us it's necessary or it becomes our choice to be completely 100 percent plant-based, then we will because we will know how. (We are prepared for the big earthquake in California with enough water and canned foods but are we prepared when we get bad news regarding our own health?) Either that or our palates will have changed a lot more because our tastes are different than when we started. I don't eat as much meat or dairy as I used to, but it's out of habit. I cook other foods I've become more accustomed to because I just enjoy them more. I enjoy eating them and not feeling so tired right after I eat too.

Think of substitutes. Butter moistens my pancakes, but coconut oil provides that same texture I'm looking for, plus the added taste of coconut. Coconut oil can be used in everything like olive oil, even in my coffee from what my friends tell me, but I'm still looking, researching, and discovering as if I'm in a lab.

I don't intend to know the proper terminology, definitions, or understanding of these diets, but this is what I can tell. I simply wanted to share how much knowledge an average person like me has on diets. I'm "college educated," I've lived in the top two most expensive cities in the U.S.—Los Angeles and New York—and I have a good career, but I'm just learning how to eat. Don't we understand how to eat or what is making us sick? If I'm found wrong, how much more wrong are so many other people? This is an important point I try to make. I'm trying to understand.

Instead of going for the sugar or butter, try eating or drinking out of a different dish or cup. Eat outside on the patio, in a comfortable chair, and see if that is just as appealing—and journal about it. Does the experience outweigh the additives to your food? Maybe not overnight, but over time of repeated tries and failures, who knows what you'll find out?

My last observation is that meat and dairy are delicacies, not everyday foods. Everyday foods are fruits, vegetables, and beans, grains like quinoa and rice, and spices. I will most likely never order a full eight-ounce steak again, but if I'm offered it, I may have a bite. It's part of being courteous, kind, and generous.

Food is so much more colorful too. I'm now posting a lot of beautiful plant-based dishes on social media with the rest of the plant-based advocates. Meat has no color and is not as beautiful. Its brown and oily look is what attracts meat lovers. I had to think about this for a minute.

Part III

THREE MONTHS LATER

So I know you're wondering, this diary sounds great, but how am I doing—how are *we* doing—three months later? Well, let me tell you the good and the bad.

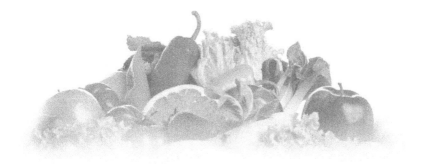

Chapter 36

The Good News

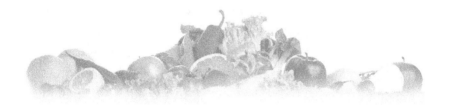

Thats right. Not buying meats and dairy products has saved us about 30 percent on our overall grocery budget. If I even add a meat or dairy product, I know I'm buying the "expensive stuff," another mind shifter. Do you want to know how to save on groceries? I have learned the simple answer. Once I cut back on meat and dairy, I was surprised at how much that fancy peanut butter was within budget. And, boy, did I find a good one. I love the chocolate almond butter; it's a bit pricey, but it's great for dessert. It's also good with apples or anything else I would normally put peanut butter on. It's nice to mix things up a bit. How many of us buy peanut butter without realizing how many other varieties of nut butter there are? It's like buying only cheddar cheese and not realizing how many other cheeses there are. We wouldn't know it, though, because any other nut butter was out of our budget, at least it was for me.

If you want to reduce your grocery bill, you can. I've done it and seen the bill. Many of us are convinced that meat and dairy products are necessary to our diets, but are they? Are we paying too much for food and gaining weight because of our beliefs handed down to us over generations? It's like discovering the true culprit wreaking havoc on our budget, let alone our waist.

Here in the United States, we believe what we are told even if it's a lie just because we've known it for so long. Maybe it's the same in other countries too. I'll explain more about that in a bit. We have believed all our lives that meat is protein, and it is, but it doesn't mean it has to be the *only* protein. With a little research, I've found other proteins such as tofu, beans, lentils, nuts, seeds, and amaranth. The highlighted foods in Google, however, are meat, fish, cheese, and yogurt. Why? Lowering your overall grocery bill will take effort and some energy, but you can do it by simply avoiding such items as meat and dairy whenever possible. We've done it, but we had to be open to other foods that have protein too.

I hear all the time that Whole Foods is so expensive and I have to agree. But guess what? It sure has gotten a lot more affordable not having a high grocery bill anymore, even with that costly peanut butter that just replaces the cost of one pound of meat. I shop at Whole Foods just to buy the extra products that are healthier, such as the chocolate almond butter I like so much with other basics, like their Italian sparkling water. I buy six one-liter sparkling waters that are $1 each in a pack at the time of writing this. The amount I paid at the register for all of this seemed enormous until I realized it was the same amount I would normally pay every week when I *recorded it* in my journal.

Richard and I stopped into Target the other day to pick up fruit and toilet paper but we also bought a t-shirt for my nephew, a couple of pizzas and two boxes each of our favorite waffles within budget. These additional items have just replaced what would have been in a previous grocery run. How is that for going on a healthy diet?

I go to Whole Foods and other specialty food stores, like the farmer's market on Third and Fairfax in Los Angeles, about once a month. One of the biggest reasons I like to go to a natural or Whole Foods store is because it's inspiring. It's comparable to hanging out at the gym even if only for a walk on the treadmill. It can be uplifting and even motivating. When I shop in a "healthy food" store, I'm shopping in an environment I wouldn't find in just any regular grocery store. Isn't this what I need when I shop for foods to eat? Isn't this what WE ALL need? To be inspired while we shop is important if we are trying to eat healthier.

Clothing stores plan everything from the way the floor is designed to the music playing to get us to buy. And, boy, do we! I didn't walk into these stores for years when I was single and on a budget. I would avoid those trigger sales floors like the plague. I would hate to want what was on sale. How does shopping make you feel? Whether we shop for clothes on a regular basis or not, we all have to buy groceries on a regular basis. Under what conditions are we buying them?

This marketing strategy also exists in ordinary grocery stores, whether we believe it or not. Wouldn't it be nice to think that shopping for groceries is different from shopping for clothes? The aisles may seem to lack nutritional items but the elevator music playing in the background has intent. Don't kid yourself. We all know why the milk has been strategically located in the back of the store, don't we? I've heard the experts talk about shopping only on the outer aisles and not in the center to stay within a healthy diet, but what good did that advice do me? Have the stores caught on to how people are shopping? They place the sugary cereals on the shelves for your kids to see and then put smaller or impulse purchases on the way to the register for you to throw in your basket. All grocery stores do this, healthy or not. They all have us pegged. They're just a store trying to get us to buy like any other type of store.

When I go to a natural or health food store, however, at least the message is loud and clear. The health food store is not subliminal at all either. These stores create an environment that reminds me of that wholesome era that once had no seat belts or talk of strange things in our Halloween candy—a time when it was safe to ride your bike for blocks without the thought of any danger. And no wonder: Martin Lindstrom, a top consultant to the biggest corporations in the U.S., a best-selling author on marketing, and a leading media contributor, writes in his book about the new and improved produce department: "By evoking farms and fresh produce, this new Pick and Prep section subconsciously evokes the ideas 'Made in the U.S.A.' and 'Healthy' and 'Community' and 'Mom' and 'Table' and 'Kitchen.'"[13] I feel better by what is promoted right at me that are as strategic as any other supermarket, but instead of slow elevator music slowing our purchasing time to buy more, there is a sentiment that gets me to purchase. Lindstrom writes, "I helped management redesign the store's fruit and produce section by using a wide variety of symbols intended to make shoppers feel 'close to the earth,' including wicker handle baskets and chalkboards on which the current market prices were scrawled in chalk."[14] The point is, wherever you shop for groceries, you'll be influenced to buy. Just *how* you'll be influenced depends on where you're buying.

And it's worked! I've bought not only the chocolate almond butter, but also coconut-flavored vinegar that is supposed to be healthier than apple cider. (Did you know how healthy apple cider is for you?) I've picked up raw, unrefined almonds that were the sweetest, best-flavored almonds I've ever had. Raw honey, flat leaf kale, salmon burgers, separately packaged, and frozen salmon strips, huge bags of frozen shrimp, a single serving size of protein shake mix, tubs of salad that don't go bad in a week, and tiny street-size corn tortillas are all just some of the products I've been *inspired* to buy. These stores introduce different kinds of cheeses from Europe with experts there waiting to help you next to the barrels of olives. Are you getting the picture?

Now I know a lot of people are saying it's different with kids or a busy lifestyle. I'm wondering, though, if we pay attention to wanting to be inspired. Kids don't have a choice. I wonder how they feel when they shop with their parents without the dozens of sugary foods on the shelves thrown at their eye level on purpose. (Did I mention how stores strategically place the products on their shelves?) In regular neighborhood stores where we might feel more humbled to shop thinking we're getting a better bargain, aren't our kids targeted to eat sugary foods at the same time?

---

13 I happened to be watching TV when I heard Lindstrom for the first time. I bought his book and sure enough, he writes about what I was trying to relay in my message in his book called *Small Data*, published by St. Martin's Press, 2016.

14 This is what Martin Lindstrom mentions in his book prior to discussing the produce section and how it would make people feel; *Small Data*: pg. 71.

In health food stores, I see vegetables lined with their bright colors made into attractive patterns instead of just piled in a heap.[15] The competition has noticed when neighborhood grocery stores are being remodeled right now. I walk into the store and notice the floors are torn out and the produce department is undergoing a facelift. I hadn't noticed the store was outdated at all. What I learn is that it's not so much a renovation because the store is getting old. It's the designs of the stores that are recreated to get customers to buy more. I can't think of a better way to attract kids to environments made up of a "Mom" and "farm" look or for those of us just looking to be inspired to eat better.

How do you feel when you walk into a specialty, natural, or health food store? Are you appalled, feel out of place, poor, or uninspired? When I talk to some people about these stores, I hear they never go in because it's too expensive. I paid attention to my emotions and what people said when I was writing this book. I couldn't help but recognize how these stores can be expensive but these stores inspire. The expensive European grocery store stretches my knowledge of what is available. I peruse the aisles to find different condiments and foods I wouldn't normally find elsewhere. Isn't this why we like to shop at Trader Joes— to find our favorite foods, delicious frozen foods or appetizers? Different grocery stores offer different kinds of food I like to buy, like the way different types of clothing stores do. It's the same concept although people look at it differently. Why?

In the past, I made friends with the butchers, who gave me all sorts of tips on how to prepare the meats I bought—even though now I feel out of touch with the butcher. The point is, if I need advice on buying vitamins or natural deodorant, which I have, a knowledgeable staff is available for those too—in a health foods grocery store. I had questions about teas and sure enough, someone pointed me to the lady "that handles the tea section." Seriously? She was helpful and knew a lot about teas all right. Regardless, I probably would be missing all these insights if I were convinced that I knew everything already.

---

15 I couldn't explain when writing this until I noticed just recently our neighborhood supermarket just renovated its produce department. They are now displaying the vegetables in the same patterns as health food stores. For example, the lettuce isn't piled at the bottom of the refrigerated shelves, they are now stacked on the higher shelves with the leaves facing outward.

Chapter 37

So Much More to Buy

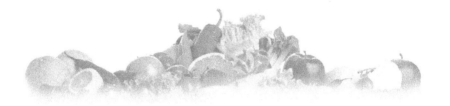

O ur grocery list is being developed with a broader range of groceries I buy. We have adapted to different staples of items to buy like plant milk and lemons but not every week. For example, I've noticed so many more choices in plant milk: soy, almond, hemp, rice, cashew, pistachio, coconut, oat, and hazelnut milk. And they may come in flavors like vanilla, plain, chocolate, light, and even seasonal flavors like peppermint. Plant milk is either cold or room temperature, making it more versatile. You probably knew that, but have you thought about how you can store cold plant milk in your fridge now and use your room temperature milk for later? I knew this too, but I hadn't *thought* about it. I can store it in my pantry longer than regular milk, but I was more caught up with wondering why we had two ways to buy milk. I like the pistachio milk and why wouldn't I? I like pistachio-flavored ice cream.

It's been hard to replace the vanilla-flavored organic creamer that froths nicely for my coffee. Like other challenges, though, I should look for a substitute that will froth just as nice as the vanilla creamer does. For now, I add only about a tablespoon of creamer to my plant milk just for it to froth nicely. The creamer tastes good, but something else out there must taste just as good because it's been the only milk that will froth for me. I like my coffee with half steamed milk and half coffee (otherwise known as "café con leche," thanks to the wonderful country of Spain where I discovered it). It's not quite a latte that has a shot of coffee, but half steamed milk and half coffee. I like to make equal parts of milk and coffee, which is my problem. Just as I no longer use sugar in my coffee, boy, do I appreciate a true good cup of coffee! My neighbor just turned me on to Americano coffee. But, wow! What a kick in the pants that is!

Because the creamer has been so hard to substitute, I've managed to use only about a tablespoon in my plant milk and steam the milk that way. It works because of the added creamer. The good news is that I've reduced the amount of dairy in my coffee to about one third of what I used to have. The bad news is that I'm still hooked on that creamer, but I know I'll find a solution eventually.

What has been challenging is finding more choices for breakfast. We have our favorite shake mix, but having shakes plain or with water is hard for both of us. I don't mind it as much, but on cold mornings it's not as pleasing to have a green shake, even with a citrus dash of lemon or lime as my girlfriend suggests. It's the psychology of having a warm drink, of course, like my old favorite, well-blended shake with warm milk, raw eggs (egg whites to be exact), cinnamon, and vanilla extract. Are the raw egg whites safe? Who knows? I never got sick but that won't be an issue anymore.

I would treat myself if my mom offered it to me, but she only makes vegetable shakes and that's what she offered me the last time. I realize I'll always be working on this. We have adopted this lifestyle and I'll be the last to say I know how to eat well because it will always be a work in progress.

We can read numerous blogs about adopting a healthier lifestyle and although this is key, they're just other perspectives. I've been able to gather information on social media, like what to have for breakfast, by searching plant-based recipes on Pinterest. I've also joined plant-based groups on Facebook for information. These resources are incredibly helpful for learning from others who are working on their plant-based diets. A great resource is the *Forks Over Knives* website (www.forksoverknives.com) with access to recipes promoted on their social media or their direct e-mail campaign delivered to my inbox. What a relief that was to find.

I learned on Pinterest about a gal who shops at Trader Joe's where she finds the gluten-free oats with quinoa, amaranth flakes, sunflower, pumpkin, hemp, flax, and chia seeds. She said it's her *and* her husband's favorite, (I guess I'm not the only one considering my spouse here). You don't know what amaranth grain is? Neither did I. It's a grain that has been around for at least eight thousand years in Mexico and Central and South America, but was banned by the Spanish conquistadors. (Those Spaniards!) Because it kept growing as a weed, however, the genetics of the grain have endured, but it wasn't until the 1970's that it was well researched (that good wholesome era when Whole Foods market was founded). Amaranth is now found primarily in health foods stores. I had never heard about it before being introduced to the gluten-free oats on Pinterest. Information like this has me continuing to learn about the abundant number of foods out there we don't even know exist. It's like discovering a whole new world.

Going back to this incredibly delicious oatmeal, which I learned about from Pinterest, I have soaked it in plant milk with fresh berries or other fruits and mixed in a hint of honey. I heat the milk and have a super-charged breakfast without the high sugar content since this oatmeal (without the honey) has about one gram of sugar. And what do most people eat? They eat oatmeal that is filled with more than nine grams of sugar (without the brown sugar) and sometimes more than that. Maybe that's small in proportion to the more than twenty-three grams of sugar in orange juice, and isn't it the sugar that is driving people to their addiction? We are finally as a culture (I think), coming to grips with the addictive nature of sugar, that it's harmful to eat, and that the effects of the cravings make it hard to stop. The good news is we can replace these foods we've always thought to be good for us with better foods!

Chapter 38

Food Storage

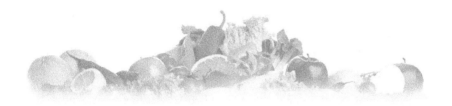

I now store a lot more products I didn't used to store. I have filled my pantry with items from plant milk to beans I didn't even think I'd keep without refrigeration. When I first bought a bag of dried beans, it would last for months, especially when I knew how long it would take to cook. I have learned to have a pantry of dried foods like beans, pasta, rice, plant milk, nuts, and grains like barley. I have found these are all essential to have in our pantry if we want to continue eating a plant-based diet. I learned I didn't need to buy four or five bags of dried beans because I used only half a bag. Was I the only one who didn't know this? Why didn't I know how to buy and measure dried beans to cook?

I store leftovers differently too. They have a different meaning these days besides something to put in the fridge to wait until it goes bad. When we think of leftovers, we typically think of something prepared from the day before. But the leftovers wouldn't have the same appeal as they did the day the food was cooked. For example, some people like cold, day-old pizza. That's fine, but I love only certain foods a day or two later, like I previously mentioned when I dealt with reheating my foods. For some reason, foods with spicy sauces are better after sitting in the refrigerator for a day or two when the spices and flavors are enriched. But this is only a small minority of foods we eat, the rest have been made certain they are not as good the next day.

This is especially true for most of the vegetarian or plant-based complete dishes I prepare. Actually, it's worse. I won't even store most completed plant-based dishes as leftovers in the fridge. I've learned to set aside a small portion of the main ingredients *before* preparing a dish. For example, if I am using anything steamed, like cauliflower, I set aside a portion of the plain steamed cauliflower, without the seasoning. Cauliflower steak is absolutely delicious. I store plain yams or sweet potatoes, asparagus, or anything else I've made in large quantities to use another day as ready-to-eat foods. Does this make sense? Instead of making the entire gluten-free pasta with sauce, I might set aside a portion of the cooked pasta without the sauce. I love to have leftover plain rice on hand in the refrigerator too. I can add rice later to a salad, fry it with other vegetables to make fried rice, learn how to make a crumble out of it to have in a taco, or add coconut milk to make a dessert. Rice is such a versatile food. It can be made in so many different ways, not just cooked in different flavors. And wouldn't you know? It says right on the package how versatile it is! I never paid attention.

Also, I'm digging more into my refrigerator than I used to. The days of sticking something in the fridge and forgetting about it are rare. I am constantly looking into storage containers as if I'm looking for something I just bought at the grocery store unopened. I'm considering buying more storage containers too. The more storage containers I can have, the better. Mine are getting pretty beaten up; I'm not sure if it's because I've had them for so long or because I'm putting them to good use. We hardly had leftovers and, if we did, they would be in the fridge for days. I'm sure we aren't the only ones who have done this either.

I stood in front of the nice-looking storage containers at the store the other day but couldn't get myself to buy any. I have to get a grip! I need to learn how to have many, if not different, types of glass storage containers I can label so I can store dried foods in the pantry and plain, cooked foods in the fridge. I have always loved how colorful the foods stored in small containers are, so this isn't foreign to me. Do you know which ones I'm talking about? Have you ever opened a home décor magazine on organization? How nice does it look to see all those colorful foods stored in glass containers? In a beautiful modern kitchen, of course.

Foods should be stored for leftovers but in separate containers from each other. Packaged foods are not the only ones that can be stored! When we think of storage containers, what are we thinking? For me, they were for leftover meals that I may or may not reheat again. We have become a culture that has relied on cans and maybe for good reason too. I've read that many people are no longer using cans because of the harmful additives in them. I watched *Top Chef* on the Food Network recently. One of the chefs competing was in a difficult situation because an ingredient was canned. I found it interesting she never used canned foods in her culinary career.

It's better to freeze than to buy in a can and I'm learning it can be done. (Hellooo, sub zero freezer!) I'm not talking about *buying* frozen foods. Once I understood that freezing could be used for everything, I have incorporated it into my habits. For example, I have a bag of cranberries left over from the holidays. I wasn't sure what to do with them so I'm freezing them. I'll come back to them later. Before, I probably would have let them go bad before deciding what to do with them. Maybe it would have never occurred to me to freeze them for later.

Why did I stare at these storage containers in the store as if they were foreign to me, as if they were a luxury? Why is that? I don't stare at cans at the grocery store, wondering whether to buy them or not and end up throwing them out.

It's as if I'm learning a whole new way of creating my pantry and refrigerator. As crazy as this sounds, it's not something we can understand unless we attempt to eat a more wholesome diet. If we went through a hyperinflation, the way Germany and many other countries have, and meat and dairy were inaccessible, I'd be prepared. From reading this book, you'll remember how to store foods although I'm not telling you how to store them. I'm giving you my account of what I learned about storing foods and incorporating a plant-based diet. I'm not one to worry about the future, but it's a good thing to know how to store dry foods and not rely on the grocer to provide the cans for us, like (again) preparing for a big earthquake in Los Angeles. We are educated on how to store water, but how about food? No one knows. It's good to know how to eat foods and not just what is fed to us. That's what I mean. Sadly, I'm sure I'm not the only one who needs to be educated on eating right.

In The China Study, Dr. T. Colin Campbell, PhD writes that the ones who are supplying the education to the medical students who eventually become our doctors and tell us what to eat are: "The Dannon Institute, Egg Nutrition Board, National Cattlemen's Beef Association, National Dairy Council, Nestle Clinical Nutrition, Wyeth-Ayerst Laboratories, Bristol-Meyers Squibb Company, Baxter Healthcare Corporation, and others [who] have all joined forces to produce a Nutrition in Medicine program and the medical Nutrition Curriculum Initiative." Do you think I'm surprised? Of course not. It's these companies who benefit from the sales of their goods sold and the doctors benefit from giving us drugs. If a doctor can't prescribe you drugs, why would they tell you they are interested in your allergy to gluten if all you need to do is avoid gluten?

Again, when I was with the Celiac Foundation group, they said it was very difficult for those with gluten sensitivities to get medical attention because there are no drugs they can prescribe you. I learned this when I told my doctor I was interested in finding out more about any gluten sensitivities I may have, but she said if I feel better by not eating gluten I should just not eat gluten because the tests were too expensive. (A doctor not prescribing expensive tests? Huh?) She then told me that it would be wiser to spend money on tests to learn more about my infertility at my age than my gluten sensitivity. Excuse me? What was funny was that I first learned about possibly having gluten sensitivity because I *couldn't* get pregnant. A friend of mine told me that it could be because of the gluten.

Do you see how this all makes sense to me? It's been like connecting the dots just like Dr. Campbell did in his China study and documentary *Forks Over Knives*. I mean, who else is going to provide education on nutrition? The farmers? Yeah, right! But what I do know is that farmers typically have a healthier lifestyle. Can you say, "farm to table?"

Dr. Campbell later writes, "You should not assume that your doctor has any more knowledge about food and its relation to health than your neighbors and coworkers."[16] And isn't this true? Isn't everyone, *including* your doctor, telling you to drink milk for good strong bones and eat steak as a good source of protein?

I once told my doctor a few years ago that I wasn't eating as good as I should because I was eating a lot of pizza but he told me pizza was not bad for me because it had enough calcium and protein in the meats and cheese. So why not eat more of it? If cheese is the culprit for me gaining weight, that clearly my body wasn't digesting thoroughly but instead storing as fat, how can that be good for me? Why wouldn't the doctor warn me to minimize it instead? Could it be because he didn't know what else to tell me I can replace the pizza with?

How's that for food storage?

---

16   Dr. T. Campbell wrote in *The China Study*, published by Benbella Books, Inc., a chapter called "Lack of Training" 328 which he finds the amount of ignorance prescribed to diabetic or people who want to lose weight "astounding." Pg. 329

Chapter 39

Filling Up Fast

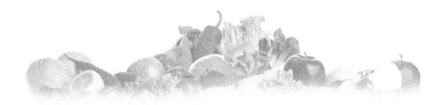

When eating only plant-based foods, be prepared to get full fast. It's almost the way you would after a hearty meal. When you eat a more healthy diet, your brain tells your stomach it's time to stop before your consciousness tells you. Let me explain. I'm sure some experts will want to correct me here, but I don't intend to be an expert. I'm just explaining how I process, so please hear me out. When I eat sugars and other non-healthy foods like a delicious cheesy hamburger, my body seems to be looking for its nutrients, because I keep eating with no sign of stopping, hence, I keep indulging *naturally*. With sugars in most of our foods, I'm constantly indulging yet telling myself I need my energy and proteins and, basically, I need to eat. This is how I've processed this information. This is how I get fat. Can anyone relate?

We only slowly get full when eating more starches, sugars, meats, and dairy because the stomach doesn't trigger the brain to stop. For example, we are eating a higher quality of protein with meats because it's more efficiently absorbed into the blood for enough protein with less, but is that necessarily *healthy*? If these proteins are absorbed so quickly that it doesn't tell my brain it's full fast enough to get me to stop eating, I'll just keep eating because I'm trained to understand that meat is the necessary (and only) protein. So I continue to clog my arteries and strain my organs even though I may be losing weight because of my smaller food portions or omission of breads but the struggle to lose weight continues. Have we not learned how to eat healthy long enough or consistently enough to know how we are eating and what we are doing to our bodies? Do we realize we have incorporated habits of indulging in foods we have decided are *good* for us even though they aren't? Are our convictions on what we've been taught on how to process it all actually be killing us?

I have to admit that sometimes after eating a healthy, plant-based meal we are full for a moment and then we're hungry again. Well, if you ask anyone who knows how to eat, we're supposed to eat five times a day. My body feels like it functions better when I've allowed it to digest the foods properly yet, I'm told to eat meat to stay satisfied until lunch or dinner. (Huh? This is what drives me crazy.)

In the beginning, I had a dessert on hand to ward off the hunger or temptations. I didn't use to buy the cookies, the pies, or the frozen turnovers for dessert to avoid the sugar and "bad habit-forming foods." Now I buy tea cookies and have one or two after dinner to suppress the sweet craving and trick my brain that I'm satisfied. I guess it's become mind over matter. Not even the chocolate chips we used to have as a dessert are what I feel so proud about now. And you know what? It works now for Richard too. I know a lot of people do this, but I'm buying the gluten-free cookies or the berries to sauté with a little port and a dash of whipped cream or I have them plain if I'm not in the mood for something fancy. I've changed my mind on how I look at desserts. What I would never have considered before I'm now considering as part of our meal. We'll have a tea cookie or piece of fruit for dessert.

Instead of indulging every day on foods that are not healthy like the meats and cheeses and avoiding desserts altogether, I'm not sure I was aware of what we were giving up when now we eat healthy all day and have a little dessert after dinner. I know a lot of people think how a plant-based diet can be so unappealing when it's actually the opposite. If we practice a healthy lifestyle and diet with just plant-based foods every day, we will eat fewer decadent burgers, desserts, and pastrami Reubens and maybe, just maybe we'll be converted. For now, these decadent and rich foods are enjoyed like water in the desert. If everyone who eats "healthy" all the time drinking their milk, eating chicken sausages for breakfast, having a strict "protein" (aka meat) diet every single day, instead of a plant-based diet, can this be why most struggle with food control too? If it's a matter of control or food portions instead of plant-based habits, is this why there always seems to be an endless cycle of confusing diets? Wouldn't an acquired (or learned) taste prove to be more effective?

Either way, this new way of eating has made me realize many of us have it backward! At least for us it's been backwards. Is this making sense? You will enjoy decadent, greasy burgers much more when you're not eating them all the time. But the only way not to eat them all the time is if you cut meat, dairy, and anything processed (which includes the "vegan" processed foods) from your everyday diet. Richard salivated over the chicken Parmesan and, with a huge grin, said, "We're having that for dinner?" It was as if we were having grandma's cooking. He was thrilled! Oh, and did I mention we can become more grateful too? I never plan on having chicken.

The rewards of making a healthy and delicious dinner after which I don't feel cramped or extremely tired are becoming the norm. It's pretty satisfying not to overeat. I like to eat to my heart's content when eating meat, but I can't say the same for a plant-based meal. Who would, right? Here's why. The truth is, it's painful to overeat a plant-based meal. I can't consume as much as I do with meat, but when I do, I'm so *painfully* full. Plant-based foods can fill me up quickly and I rarely have seconds. It's not because I don't like it or because I'm trying to lose weight; I *know* what it feels like. It's not that I feel sick, rather, it's as if someone punched me in the stomach when I overeat a plant-based dish. I can't have too much stir-fry, cauliflower, vegetable tacos, or broccoli salad. I know not to eat more than I should but I can only describe why. It's hard to explain. Maybe seeing more documentaries and reviewing the *Forks Over Knives* movie again will help me understand why we are full sooner with eating vegetables because after all, there is an explanation in the movie. All I can say is there is a difference.

Chapter 40

Learning to Cook

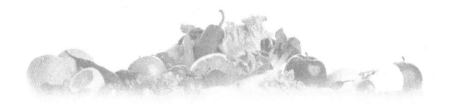

I f you are going to try to incorporate a plant-based diet or any type of "healthy" lifestyle, you will have to know how to cook. Period. Don't kid yourself.

I love to cook, but changing one's eating habits may be very difficult for those who don't cook. Unless you plan to hire a chef, have food delivered, or have another person in your home cook for you, eating a whole food, plant-based diet will be more difficult for you than it already is if you don't learn how to cook. Preparing dinner as if it was a Broadway show is no longer the norm in our home anymore. I used to prepare a roast, hamburgers, and spaghetti and meatballs with my eyes closed, fry the chicken in a deep fryer we received as a wedding gift and even went so far as to brine short ribs in wine. I did this as if it were part of a well-practiced musical play I would perform like a pro. Now that I consistently cook differently, it's more like an operation in a surgical room. I'm focused on the chemistry of it and praying for the best.

Sometimes it doesn't come out and other times it's beautiful and great tasting. It's frustrating, though.

Maybe this is why people have every excuse in the world for not attempting this lifestyle: it's hard. On the other hand, when I do get it right, the discipline is the same as being on a golf course. After so many bad swings, if I drive the ball more than a hundred feet straight on the fairway, followed by an oh-so-gentle ping sound at the end of my club, it's pure bliss! It's all the same discipline to me. If you could care less about these types of victories, this won't be a fun lifestyle. Trust me. Are there people, especially women, who think I'm either nuts or will lose interest in golf over time? Of course. The same story applies when eating a plant-based diet.

I've learned it gets tiring. You want to break out with the eggs and cheese and wrap it around a flour tortilla. You know what I do when I'm tempted? I just do it! If I can't take it anymore and I'm out of energy and enthusiasm, I go for it. When I give in, I can only say it never feels good, especially when I'm writing this book on changing my eating habits! But I'm emotionally or physically drained when I give in because I'm reminded how much I get tired after decadent melted cheese on anything. That may be why it's becoming less and less tempting. When I binge, I feel guilty, bloated, sick, or lethargic, but mostly lethargic. Then I'm reminded that the thrill is gone. It's like getting older; you can only take so many late nights of partying before the hangover isn't worth it anymore. So why are you upset that you binged? Just do it already! You'll either get tired of the thrill or succumb to it forever.

I like to keep things simple. "If it doesn't grow in the ground or can be plucked off a tree," as an herbalist in Hawaii told me, it's probably not helping my overall health. By sticking to a plant-based diet, I'm getting it. I've agreed and this has become my take on it. It's not what most people would think. Most people who've picked up this book might want to know how I would write about how I couldn't eat this or "Oh, I can't eat that." Even the Bible says that anything that commands you, "Do not handle! Do not taste! Do not touch! . . . are all destined to perish with use because they are based on human commands and teachings."[17] Without sounding spiritual, it is human nature to try and control our discipline. Diet programs have benefited immensely because we naturally have little control over our own choices. This is why, for most diet programs, there is always an eating regimen to follow.

Eating healthy should be a habit. I like to think we have adopted *knowing* what is good and what isn't from *experience*. Having knowledge of what is good for me will last through the long haul, not just while I'm on a diet. I now know what to research when I cook. If you want to live healthier, feel better, and even lose weight, I'm afraid there's no way around not learning how to cook or at least prepare food for yourself. Many people choose popular diets because they don't know *what* to cook. How can we be such an educated culture, probably the most educated in history, and yet we are reverting to not being educated on how to feed ourselves?

If you don't want to believe me, then at least take Anthony Bourdain's perspective; he's a culinary chef, host of CNN's *Parts Unknown*, author, father, husband, and world traveler. In one of his books, *Medium Raw*, he writes that learning how to cook in grade school needs to be reintroduced the way we need to learn hygiene (and that's all I'm going to say about that). I agree with his philosophy. I always wondered how, when basic cooking skills were being taught as a fundamental skill, it was also branded as a course popular for girls. Bourdain has a great explanation for how it was institutionalized as a social responsibility in which women "were indoctrinated with the belief that cooking was one of the essential skill sets for responsible citizenry—or, more to the point, useful housewifery."[18]

I know what happened. Home economics was removed and us girls were put in woodshop that not only we resented but I wonder if it was a resentful move against the feminist movement. While the women protested, no one was paying attention to the fact that an education on how to cook was eliminated, complete with an education on nutrition. Sure, there was a culture class with more young

---

17 I'm not trying to get spiritual here, but if it's quoted in the Bible as a human truth, I'm the type to take it as the truth. Colossians 2:21-22

18 Anthony Bourdain explains how our culture may have depreciated the virtue of such a fundamental skill in *Medium Raw*. Published by Harper Collins, pg. 60.

women not wanting the stigma of being a homemaker anymore. We want to be treated not just equal but respected and teaching us how to cook so that we can cook for our *family* I can see as an insult. Doesn't *everyone* need to know how to cook the way we all need to know how to handle our finances?

Women want to be known for making more of an impact instead of on a man and why not? However, is the punishment for the way things were handled with home economics being eliminated, ignorance? Has the result of not requiring boys to take home economics been destructive to our overall health statistics?

Bourdain goes on to say, and rightly so, "By the end of the 60s, *nobody* was cooking . . . no one even remembered *how*."[19] And here is where he brilliantly suggests what I'm trying to suggest, that our generation should spearhead the revival of a lost art if not a survival skill. I agree that we should all know how to chop an onion, dice, mince, and slice. We should all know how to handle a knife, a mandoline and a *Pampered Chef* chopper. Do we even know how to sharpen a knife and learn its maintenance so we don't cut ourselves? Who doesn't know someone who hasn't? (How many of us have cut ourselves with a kitchen knife than a woodshop tool?) It would be good for everyone to know how to make basic vinaigrettes and even shop for produce by knowing what is in season and what is ripe. I sure would have in my early twenties!

I was amazed at finding the bones and meat pieces at a farmer's market at such a low price and then realized it was for chicken stock. I was well past forty when I realized we could buy chicken pieces this way. Why? Bourdain says we should all know what to do with bones, but I didn't even know they were sold like that. I didn't learn about making stock out of leftover roasted chicken until well into my thirties. Is it because I'm from a more suburban area? I agree that we should know how to make soups to save money. We all need to learn that at some point in our lives. I would agree that not only would it have been wise for me to learn when I was in my twenties, single, and on a budget, I would have learned how to eat a lot healthier living on a budget too. How many times do we say we can't afford to eat healthier?

---

19 I have to say that in the 80's, it wasn't even up for discussion, but who else can remember cooking in our culture during that time other than Anthony Bourdain? *Medium Raw*, pg. 61.

I worked with a gal who didn't come in one day because she said she got food poisoning. I totally believed it. She looked awful! She said the doctor told her she probably didn't cook her chicken thoroughly the night before. "Every citizen should know how to throw a piece of meat in the oven without the expectation that they might roast it to somewhere in the neighborhood of desired doneness—without a thermometer."[20]

We all need to know how to cook, both men and women. This shouldn't be a discussion of chivalry vs. feminism. Isn't it more a parent and child responsibility: part of our humanity responsibility of existing? Our very lives depend on it. As I mentioned earlier, count yourself lucky if you have someone to cook for you. My husband is lucky he found someone who likes to cook because he doesn't know how. When we got married, he didn't even know how to fry an egg. I kid you not. Apparently, I *do* know those who don't know how to cook and some who don't know how to cook meat too. We took beautiful, seasoned boxed steaks to a friend's house for dinner years ago and I maniacally stopped all production in the kitchen when they were about to be submerged in water for rinsing. It was bad enough we didn't have wine with it that night, but rinsing a beautifully prepared seasoned steak? I protested loudly!

Today, we now are mesmerized with cooking shows and chefs becoming TV celebrities because of their introduction to simple recipes we should have already learned in cooking a basic class.

As Bourdain ends this topic of learning basic skills on how to cook, so will I. He says, "Why can we not do this? There is no reason in the world. Let us then go forward. With vigor."[21]

---

20 Anthony Bourdain addresses this issue better than I could have, especially as a well-known chef, someone who has made a living serving most likely the most educated. *Medium Raw*, pg. 63.

21 Anthony Bourdain's last word on the virtue of cooking—all excerpts taken from the chapter titled "Virtue." *Medium Raw*, pg. 64.

Chapter 41

Home Ec

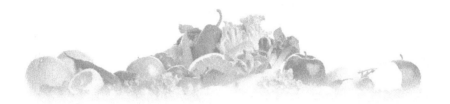

We no longer have to go to the bookstore or the library, although I'm certainly not knocking that idea. These are the best places to hang out where I can feel as if I'm among a deep and wide knowledge of anything I want to know. However, we also have the bookshelves of every library in the world practically at our fingertips unless we are the curmudgeons who still believe we don't need computers. I didn't think so.

I agree with Anthony Bourdain in that we need to go back to the basics and teach our children to cook, starting in middle school. Instead of the woodshop and drafting classes I had to endure with who knows what else they substituted that for, we need to teach our kids not just how to eat but how to cook. It was for good intentions to try to get students to learn how to function in society, but this is the age where young kids need to learn how to cook. Let's start there. Yes, at one time home economics (aka home ec) class was taken primarily by girls and had a stigma with it too. I agree. The thought of my college friend saying she wanted to take a home ec class to learn how to cook almost had me disown a non-feminist friend on the spot. How could someone like me, "a journalism major," hang out with someone who took home economics? College was for the "career oriented." Well, shame on me. Today, not many people know how to cook and, when we don't know how to cook, we don't know how to eat. It's plain and simple.

The *Boston Globe* correspondent Ruth Graham wrote an article that inspired writers and investigative journalists (whom I find more authoritative on this subject than myself) to talk about how important it was to bring back home economics that I found very interesting.

"Almost a third of Americans under age 19 are now overweight or obese, habituated to a diet of cheap processed food,"[22] a statistic we would probably all agree with. What was astounding, however, were the quotes Graham found that I have to add here to conclude in my findings. Understand that I have come to these conclusions because of what I read in my own journal. What these researchers are finding just happened to be related to what I found.

Graham includes in her article a statement by Helen Zoe Veit, a historian who challenged the status quo by stating how important home ec was to handling the obesity problems rather than just wearing a fancy apron. She said, "A beautiful way to start solving this problem would be to get more people cooking. We have a blueprint of how to do this, and it's through home economics."[23] Bingo. It looked like I had a case. However, I wonder if these woman's ideals of how we can make a change were simply ignored with a complete action of wiping the entire course out.

But let's not stop there. Graham also mentions an argument by an investigative journalist, Michael Moss, who wrote a book titled *Salt, Sugar, Fat* that became a best seller. Moss argued that major companies had a foothold over Americans and profited off the fast and heavily processed foods. (No kidding!) He also wanted to see home economics brought back in such a way that students would

---

22 I found this article when I researched on the Internet whether it's home ed (for home education) or home ec (for home economics). This article was written by Ruth Graham, a Boston Globe Correspondent in an online article called *Bring Back Home ec!* Oct. 13, 2013.

23 We have curriculums for healthier diets and it's in the very curriculum that can be more accomplished in schools. Ruth Graham, *Bring Back Home ec!* Boston Globe Correspondent, Oct. 13, 2013.

recognize the name and perhaps be brought back to the age level where more students would grasp it. He states, "The decline of home economics is a huge part of the shift in this country to mindless eating."[24] So now men are on board?

I like Bourdain's idea of bringing back the lessons of how to prepare a simple dish like cooking an egg, but I wasn't prepared for what I found online when I researched the movement to bring back home ec. I felt I was making assumptions from my experience by concluding that no one knew how to cook. Little did I know this had been up for discussion for some time. Bourdain's recommendations for how to clean and sharpen a knife, to how to bake simple dishes, resonated with me because I'm not only a fan of his shows and books but my findings were the same. It turns out I'm not the only one tooting my horn.

We argue that our children are not learning how to eat anymore because they don't know how to cook, and we share our statistics with each other and with the world. Meanwhile, the diet business is accelerating into an economy of billions of dollars to teach people how to eat, how to cook, and how to count their calories. So who's complaining? I too used to sell a dietary supplement myself!

It's a challenge to eat in a way that could make me live longer and healthier and be happier with myself. It has showed me we are living in a crisis of not just hunger around the world, but also a common eating disorder. We have been like sheep going to the slaughter house being fed foods that go beyond just making us fat, they are addictive and are not only sold to us but are being labeled as "good" for us. The foods we are eating are slowly making us sick, possibly feeding cancerous cells within our bodies we are unaware of that only take the lives of our family and friends. Culturally, we are hungry for more entertainment because our energy to think and be active slowly comes to a halt as we lie on our couches all evening from malnutrition that lends itself to brain fog.

We are at war with the philosophies of Obamacare yet savor how Michelle Obama raps with the rappers about how to eat better. We complain about the costs of medical care, but we are convinced we need the foods that harm our bodies. And it's our convictions that are leading us to medication and surgeries. I don't know why I've had the same problem for years and neither do the doctors.

24   If children don't start learning how to eat, they are vulnerable to generations that don't know how to eat. Ruth Graham quotes Michael Moss's book in *Bring Back Home ec!* Boston Globe Correspondent, Oct. 13, 2013.

What they know is that I'll most likely need medication for a very long time. That is always the answer, but is it?

We may need to teach our kids how to cook and bring home ec back to our schools if we're ever going to change. If we can't feed ourselves, who will? The idea of chefs entering the business of culinary education has gained traction as well as popularity, thanks to television channels such as the Food Network, Travel Channel and of course, CNN. It's nice to see TV programs on how even young children are competing to be the best chef, but are we acknowledging this concept and taking it to the classrooms?

How can meat be a luxury of the wealthy yet is as common as walking into a fast food chain and ordering it with cheese? Whether it's ground meat or steak, we are ambitious to eat meat. It's as if our population has been brain washed into believing we need milk and eggs as much as we need sleep (and, boy, have I heard this over and over again by simply mentioning that we are avoiding meat). They ask questions from, "How does that work?" to "What do you eat on a *normal* day?" to "What about your protein?" When I don't order eggs at a restaurant, I'm asked, "Don't you want your protein?" I have to say, it didn't take every part of me not to order it either. I have learned I can eat protein in so many other foods, although I can still enjoy eggs for Easter brunch, but not every time I want to sit down and have breakfast.

We have been trained to drink dairy for calcium and eat meat for protein for as long as I can remember. My generation has been born on this concept. Chase Chandler, a financial advisor who does extensive studies on human behavior when it comes to our choices, simply writes in one of his books that we easily revert to what we've been taught for years. I agree in that, if we try something new, we may go back to what we were told even if it was a lie. In his book, *The Wealthy Family,* he writes, "The natural reaction is to revert to our previous behaviors and habits, to what we know."[25] And in the case of our eating habits, if we've been taught to eat our meat and dairy for years, we'll just keep reverting back to these eating habits again and again as we struggle with our weight and health, inherent in not eating well.

---

25 *The Wealthy Family* is a book written by Chase Chandler who is a non-conformist financial advisor.

The challenge for Richard and I is not to go back to our old eating habits. We have to evaluate the information, process it, experiment with it, practice it, and come to our own conclusions. I understand this is not for everyone. Who wants to put themselves in something as challenging as this?

The key is teaching this process to kids: how to cook vegetables and make soups and how to buy fruits and vegetables. We need to experiment with eating the right foods. Our parents who told us what to eat may not have known better either; they passed on what they were told. Not only that, but our generation bridged the gap from cooking from scratch to microwave dinners and fast-food chains. Nothing is shameful about that—or about having to go from one income to two or finding easier and more efficient ways to raise kids. What is shameful is that, culturally, we take basic fundamental skills of learning how to feed ourselves and make it a political warfare about who was supposed to do it. Who was supposed to lead this, or who is responsible for what happened? I think of that song by The Rolling Stones in which Mick Jagger sings about Kennedy's death: "After all, it was you and me." We are all guilty of killing the basic fundamentals of cooking in our culture because we argued over whose job it was, and if you read Anthony Bourdain's *Kitchen Confidential,* you'll learn that it was the immigrants who came over and found work in something no one here wanted to do nor knew how.

The good news is that instead of trying to figure out which kind of eggs to order, such as brown or white, caged or organic, I don't have them anymore. I'm like the housewife who throws in the towel and says, "I just don't have to cook them anymore!"

Chapter 42
Reverse Psychology

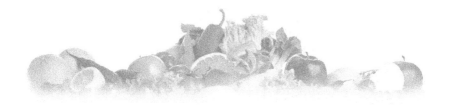

If we don't like to eat foods that remind us of what is inedible, like how spaghetti squash reminds my husband of waxed string, some vegetables remind me of something I love that will keep me trying to eat it that way even though I consistently don't like it. For me, spaghetti squash reminds me of hash browns even though it never comes out. When I scrape the yellow squash out, the texture is denser than pasta and, with it being yellow in color; I can almost see it turn crispy in the pan. I keep researching ways to eat fried spaghetti squash even though I can find a number of ways to eat it like spaghetti with meat sauce. I'd much prefer to find a way to eat it like hash browns even though it doesn't taste the same as nice, crispy hash browns but I'll still keep trying even though I've nearly given up. I was disappointed when I tried to make fritters out of this stringy squash, but it didn't come out. I might have to give up on the whole thing.

This is probably why, as it turns out, I'm not a big fan of spaghetti squash. Even though it tastes good with marinara sauce, psychologically, it should be hash browns. Therefore, I don't buy this squash as much.

I admit I'm having a hard time using regular water in my shakes too. Many healthy people use water and maybe add lime. But I've been drinking smoothies for more than twenty years and the closest thing I've used to water is aloe vera juice or coconut water with the pulp. I might try it with only water, but I'll have to start slow. I started using milk, of course, and then juice for years, but adding water sounds as if it would make it taste bland. I may wait for the weather to warm up. That will be a tough one. Smoothies have always had juice and, somehow, I have to overcome this; coconut water for now may do—at least for now.

I know I'm convinced that if I cook with turnips they will be as bland as they look. I avoid fresh beets, thinking they will stain my blouse, even though that's never happened. My mother swears by them though. I've acquired a taste to parsnips probably because they resemble carrots, but I somehow mistake them for tasting like jicama by not buying them sometimes. I start to grab the Napa cabbage, but without an Asian dish in mind, I go for the regular cabbage. I dumped iceberg lettuce a few years ago because it didn't have the nutrients other salad greens had, such as spinach and romaine lettuce, but it shouldn't have been a reason to never buy it anymore.

Richard and I haven't changed completely but we have changed and are continuing to change. That is the bottom line. It's not the Paleo diet, the gluten-free diet, the Atkins or the South Beach diet, or the vegan-vegetarian-pescatarian diet that will transform our lives overnight with the decision to start on Monday. I'm convinced it's in trying to eat a basic, plant-based diet that will help us to eat healthy overall by training our palate.

Years ago, we watched a movie called *Food Inc.* that began our curious journey to learn more about the foods we eat. We went from 1 percent milk to fat free milk to organic milk. Now we don't even drink milk. We went from never thinking about the Whole Foods market to making it a date on a Friday night and finding the best burger for five bucks. They have a wine-tasting section that opens sometimes for sampling too. Who would argue? Before we started our new lifestyle, we noticed the well-cut, fresh meats such as the smoked lamb shank we bought for twenty bucks. We shared this with a bottle of wine and considered it a cheap date. The Pasadena store has a lounge where customers may eat and drink wine as the store's way to bring in customers and buy their inventory. It would work for us but that store isn't near us.

Or how about the one-pound smoked ribs for about ten bucks that were on sale every Friday between 4 and 7 p.m.? I was making dinner when Richard said he had to run down to pick up these ribs for an "appetizer." Although we learned about the delicious offerings at Whole Foods, we hardly eat like this anymore. And it's not because the Whole Foods market is expensive! If anything, we have eaten like royalty for a lot cheaper than in a fancy restaurant and Los Angeles has plenty of expensive restaurants to choose from.

If it wasn't for the convincing documentary *Forks Over Knives*, though, we would never have learned how foods can heal our ailments. It's the whole food, plant-based diet that eliminated all the hype, the irrational conclusions, the special packaging, and the extra reading I had to do at the grocery store—in short, it was simple enough to follow. If the study was to convince the audience how a lot of diseases can be controlled with diet and eliminate all the drugs diabetics have to take every day, it was convincing.

The China Study on medication was also convincing. My doctor told me I might have to be on a medication for who knows how long and take all kinds of uncomfortable tests. This was enough motivation for me to find an alternative in naturally healing foods and *The China Study* helped to process this information because it was simple and validating. There certainly is an argument throughout the whole book.

Although I've always liked the homeopathic healing process better, I know not everyone is like this too. When it comes to change, however, I think we're all the same. I'm like many people who think, "If it doesn't kill me, I'll go for it!" We only live once! I would never turn down a Dodger dog at Dodgers stadium. (I think.) But here is where my journal comes in. I'm like all those others who tried eating differently, yet were left confused. I wrote this journal as a way for others who may need to see what I've discovered and be convinced we might be on to something.

Chapter 43

Thinking Differently

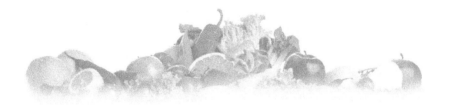

When eating out, we're happy sharing an appetizer and an entrée with wine and dessert, and this is the norm for many people, but not necessarily for us. Richard took me out for my birthday at one of our favorite restaurants and neither one of us was willing to share any appetizer, entrée, or even dessert. I wanted what I wanted, and so did he, and neither of us was going to budge. I suggested we take a bottle of wine to save paying a corkage fee. Richard refused because he thought he wasn't up for drinking that much (having a plant-based mind?). But when he sat down, he ordered the bottle of wine (having Richard's mind).

When we ordered, I wasn't going to give up trying the arugula salad with persimmons. I wanted to explore that fruit, especially when my parents had raved about it when I wasn't used to it. How could I not try it at a fancy restaurant where it's prepared uniquely? Richard, on the other hand, never gives up having a Caesar salad. He wanted the veal in exchange for a steak he probably thought about, and I was only in the mood for fish if we were indulging. He wanted the apple pie. With the red wine left over, I wasn't about to ruin this pairing, so how could I turn down the rare opportunity with the chocolate flourless cake?

Well, we were over-stuffed and over budget even with our discount. We were like priests after lent. Although we had acquired a taste for good foods, the constraints of our habits were taken over by our old habits. And that happens. Especially in the first few weeks, old habits won't be won overnight.

We couldn't complain of overeating this holiday season (and, trust me, there was plenty to be had), but the amount of eating threw my husband for a spin. He acquired a fever that reminded me of the psychological effects our environment has on our psyche. When I was a child, our family went into Mexico and, when we crossed the border, I was struck with the border town's smell of exhausts, dirt roads, and being in unknown territory that threw my young body for a spin. I had a fever and was just nauseous. My parents tried giving me something to eat but I didn't want any of it. I was told I had the flu. Richard too, became nauseous and ran a fever on the last day of our holiday break. I knew it could have been from indulging in rich foods for a few days that weren't in our normal diet, but we dealt with it as if it were the flu. Back at home, he was fine and ready to eat healthy again the way I probably was when we crossed back into the United States when I was young. When we returned to the United States, I was hungry for McDonald's again.

I think the psychology of this whole process has kept my husband from overeating and that in and of itself makes trying this extreme way of eating—okay, *healthy lifestyle*—worthwhile. The process of transitioning to eating healthier is psychological. And no doubt that's what this has been for us. It's as if Richard and I have gone back to the dark ages and have adopted eating barley, wheat, and vegetables from the earth the way it was intended thousands of years ago and, like the same humans we were back then, we have adjusted. (And, yes, humans have always consumed meat, but it was also a sign of wealth, wasn't it?) It's as if our bodies are adjusting in a good way and experiencing something different from foods rich in meat and dairy. My body certainly doesn't feel heavy anymore. I'm also not that dependent on coffee to keep me going. It's like learning how to be happy and going back to being unhappy just doesn't do it for us anymore.

Right now, however, we are low on groceries. I've been going a bit more infrequently to the grocery store until we're almost out of everything. My husband broke down and bought eggs, but guess what? He only bought a half dozen. Was he kidding? I can't remember how many eggs he ate, but all we had in the fridge were eggs and soy chorizo (not necessarily a whole plant food). But I thought, why not? I'll eat those eggs and decided to use two. I usually eat only one, but I was hungry from eating a smaller portion at dinner last night. My mind reset itself and I told myself, "Just do it. What will eating two eggs hurt?" (Well, what can it?) So I cooked both eggs, had a few small tacos, and felt completely satisfied until I started feeling fatigued! It's as if I were being punished for doing something I wasn't supposed to do, never mind the feeling of guilt. I didn't feel bad for having the egg like probably most who cheat on their diet. I felt mad at myself because now I was fatigued and I had work to do and with that, the few dozen eggs Richard bought have been in the fridge for a couple of weeks.

We were thinking differently because we were able to change our eating habits when we relied on our palate and how we feel instead of trying to control it. The thought of how we'll feel after eating like this helped us manage our food portions. I have found that when people have convictions of what to eat, it becomes a matter of what foods to eat. Dr. Campbell suggests, "…following this diet requires a radical shift in your thinking about food…if you are curious about these findings but know in your heart that you will never be able to give up meat—then I know that no amount of talk will ever convince you to change your mind."[26]

In studying my journal, I wonder if it's the food Richard and I have an opinion on that tells us what to eat. We are beginning to be convinced meat and dairy are not good for us by the way we feel, but in talking with others, I hear people feel they need meat to *be* better. Nothing could change their belief but trial and error; experience. When people eat meat every day or even every other day, is this healthy? If we are uncompromising on the foods that kill us, what diet could help us? In other words, if we are choosing meat over vegetables or believe meat is just as healthy for us *as* vegetables, are we eating to cure

---

26 T. Colin Campbell Ph.D describes in chapter 12 "How To Eat" in *The China Study,* 244

sicknesses, or are we sick because of what we are eating? Managing our weight is only the beginning.

I have found the most powerful way to manage our eating is not only to change our eating habits, but also to change our minds. Richard and I are evolving in how we eat by how we think. We have changed our minds by adopting the idea that eating is a way of healing and not just to satisfy our appetites. We never considered what we ate bad, but we would often be teased for eating so unhealthy, and for good reason. We love golf and what else is there to eat but a warm breakfast burrito on the first tee or a fried hot dog in a warm bun on the 9th tee? Even though we've succumbed to the ham and cheese instead, is that even a healthier choice by comparison? Today it wouldn't be.

We've become so much more disciplined and strict in our eating habits that we might snub the same people who teased us whose eating habits might now be worse than ours were. I was so embarrassed one time when we took donuts to church and Richard couldn't give them away. Finally, someone asked him, "Are you nuts? Why are you eating that stuff?" We liked treating ourselves to donuts before church, and who doesn't like coffee and donuts? (For some, it's like beer and chips or peanut butter and jam.) Richard had me hooked on ham and cheese croissants. We didn't do this all the time, but the truth is we did it often.

The last time we stopped for a ham and cheese croissant, I bought him chocolate milk. He said it was the first milk he'd had in months! I felt bad for giving it to him. Instead, we are getting in the habit of having potatoes or fruit in the morning before heading out the door or maybe indulging ourselves by splitting a breakfast burrito on the way to church. (It's our way of cheating on our diet.) It's these sorts of things we haven't conquered—but not without feeling that we still need to. And it's not so much because we need to be more determined or have more self-control. We need to change our minds in how we look at it. We need to learn more of what is out there. From discovery, I know many other choices await us.

Chapter 44

Indulging

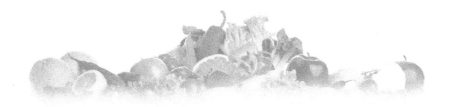

C heating on eggs or meat has become one of our big cheats these days. From time to time, we would indulge in a greasy burger, fries, and a shake; the same is true now for splitting a corned beef Reuben sandwich at the farmer's market. When Richard saw me coming home with it, he said, "Food!" as if he's been starved for days. What we consider cheating is not necessarily the chocolate cake or the butter cream pies. We are now cheating on the same foods we ate regularly. We used to eat eggs, cow's milk, ground turkey, ground steak, chicken sausage, breakfast sausage, summer sausage, pork sausage, pork chorizo, yogurt, butter, sour cream, coffee creamer, pork chops (the bone-in kind? Yes, those), steak, pork ribs, chicken, lamb, bacon, ham-and-cheese breakfast burritos, cheddar, Parmesan, jack, Cotija, mozzarella, goat and brie cheeses, meatless crumbles, vegan hot dogs, fish, shrimp, salmon burgers, and the like. We always had these foods in our fridge. Now these are the foods we treat ourselves with on the weekend, with a glass of wine or dinner out with friends or family. They are more like a delicacy. All of it.

Now that we are more focused on eating plant-based foods, we know what we need to be eating. We're in our mid-forties with no serious health issues as I'm writing this, and we indulge every once in a while. I'll surprise Richard with orange chicken with rice and a salad, or we'll have a little steak with family but in very small sizes (you know, the size of a deck of cards) and, yes, with a bottle of wine. Most of the week is purely plant-based.

I'm hoping the less we indulge, the less we'll want to, but we have yet to experience no cravings. We still indulge ourselves on a burger or filet mignon and lobster at a family gathering during the holidays. Last week while on a weekend getaway, we were at a steakhouse ordering appetizers and, without flinching, we agreed to enjoy our time away and each indulged on a burger from their bar menu. It was one of those smaller burgers, but it was perfect. Steakhouses typically offer a fantastic gourmet burger sometimes found on the bar menu and, with a glass of wine and fries, we relished it.

I have found eating like this to be the norm for a lot of folks, though. I know it used to be for us even though we often tried to tell ourselves we knew better. I would have a burger "this one time," not realizing I'd already had meat a few times in the past week. And isn't the ground meat the most harmful? It's not the lettuce, tomato, and onions that is necessarily bad, it's the ground beef that is the killer. Unless we think we need meat for protein, then the vicious cycle just continues.

I've heard it's our blood type, our genetics, and our background—where we're from that will tell us how or why we eat. I have a book on blood types that has helped me understand what my blood type is in order to eat the right foods. The truth is, genetically, my body is prone to arthritis from former generations, including my mom and grandmother, who have endured having it. This is why I abstain from gluten as much as I can. I've heard that if your family comes from the sea, though, you're more likely to eat fish than if your family is from the prairies where you're more prone to eat meat. Either way, though, I always knew eating fruits and vegetables has always been healthier. Richard and I are just changing the way we look at indulging our appetites and cravings, and that is everything.

Chapter 45

The Subconscious Mind

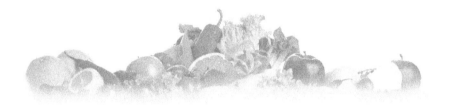

We make New Year's resolutions even if just subconsciously. However, it's much more than the choices we make. I wanted to choose a healthier diet, but I also wanted to be transformed. Early in the year, I told my husband I wanted to eat less and spend less. I wasn't sure how that would happen or even what it would look like until eight months later when we watched *Forks Over Knives* for the second time and realized we needed to be more radical in our *habits*. What we didn't realize was that it hit deep in our subconscious. Maybe because we had considered spending and eating less, something about this documentary challenged us to try it. I ponder about the power our brain has over our entire body. I'm not a scientist, but I once heard our subconscious is like an ant controlling an elephant. I have experienced how this process has controlled the way I have thought about eating.

With eating differently—which came with the painful disciplines of failure day after day—it was almost as if Richard wanted to be able to control something.

If we were going to do this, he would control his exercise. So Richard began to run again. He would come in and mention how many laps he did and whether he accomplished his goal. I was busy in the kitchen like a mad scientist and he was running a few laps in a small park behind our building. It was as if our subconscious minds were at work more than we knew what we were succumbing to. And this is what we surrendered to—nearly eleven months after deciding to eat less and spend less, we were eating a lot less and spending less. I didn't know what it looked like when I made that resolution, but something told me we were spending too much just for the two of us also.

We are adopting a diet of foods that can cure diabetes and heart disease and reverse genetically damaging health issues like high blood pressure. I don't know about you, but this looks like a fountain of youth. Why *wouldn't* we want to learn how to eat this way? Well, I can only conclude that we are a culture of guilty pleasures from the way we eat to the way we spend, even if it will cost us our lives. If we are absolutely confident that meat is necessary even though there are nutritional experts, some doctors, but, most importantly, scientists who say otherwise, who else can stop us?

My chiropractor would always warn me of the damaging effects of red meat. He said red meat produces acid that breaks down the cartilage. In more recent studies, I found it's the cow's milk that degenerates the cartilage in arthritis. "When susceptible people put all these foreign animal proteins in their bodies, one of 2 things may happen, when we nibble on the cartilage at the end of a chicken's leg, our immune system may react to these foreign cartilage proteins by producing anti-cartilage antibodies that may get confused and start attacking our own cartilage. That's what they mean by 'Meat-Induced Joint Attacks.' The other possibility is that even if there is no cross reactivity confusion, the immune complex that is formed by the meat proteins or antibodies may migrate over to the joints and trigger inflammation that way."[27] It's the "proteins" that we are proud to add to our diets but that also attack the cartilage at the joints.

And while the animal proteins break down my cartilage, bread can also be the cause of inflammation. According to Rochelle Rosian, MD, a rheumatologist

---

27   Michael Greger, M.D. is a New York Times bestselling author who explains this on one of his numerous videos on nutrition. His videos can be found on www.nutritionfacts.org, a highly viewed website on nutrition.

at Cleveland Clinic, "We know that certain foods are pro-inflammatory and that includes gluten-containing grains and the thousands of foods made from them. When some, but not all, people with celiac disease or gluten sensitivity eliminate these from their diet, they find their arthritis improves."[28]

I feel it in my left thumb and in my neck when I eat a lot of bread, as I mentioned earlier. Here is the kicker, though. I wouldn't know what was happening overall if I wasn't paying attention to what I've been advised and sometimes I still don't. I don't automatically feel the effects of weak joints. Over time, as I mature, however, my joints could start to ache and when the pain becomes too unbearable, I'll see a doctor. When I see a doctor, the damage is already done. Then it's surgery. Well, no, thank you. I'd like to avoid that for as long as I can. My mother is now fretting that, when she is finally able to visit Italy, she might have to set that trip aside for knee surgery. Do you think I see the warning signs? Let me tell you, these are not the choices I'd like to have if I can help it.

Living in a capitalistic society brings tremendous freedoms, but self-interest groups can easily capitalize on promoting the foods we eat. However, responsibility is also expected in a society run by the bourgeois of industrialism. As the wealthy have huge responsibilities, so do its citizens. The party will only last as long as the person is able to manage their wealth, and this goes for how we have been feeding ourselves too. Let's not make the mistake of thinking that living in a culture like Willy Wonka's chocolate factory for days on end doesn't have a price. It's a price for living and swimming in chocolate milk every day. Unless you are Charlie Bucket who passes Willy Wonka's moral test, be prepared to pay the price.

When I started writing down everything, little did I know what I would accomplish other than this book. The goal was to track my thinking and take note of what I liked. But from writing this journal, I gained different convictions. I also had a lot of questions but, regardless, I was reducing our grocery bill. I was able to realize a goal and piece together a puzzle that linked our spending habits for groceries.

---

28   Dr. Rosian was quoted in the Arthritis Foundation website at www.arthritis.org under *The Connection Between Gluten and Arthritis* tab.

If grocery stores are trying to inspire us to shop more responsibly, why is it getting such a bad rap? If they're over-charging in error, are they under-charging too? Is Trader Joe's the healthy alternative when I'm buying everything frozen and already packaged? Why is it so much easier to get everything under one roof at the regular grocery store? It's more convenient not to have to visit many other stores to get the items I need when I go grocery shopping at the local neighborhood store. Is it cost effective to buy products that will last us six months to a year? My mind has been subconsciously processing all of this.

If a physician AND a professor of nutritional biochemistry both examine their studies in *Forks Over Knives,* who are not linked with any food companies profiting from the foods they are promoting and who both agree that diseases can be reversed with diet, why wouldn't we try it? Why wouldn't we examine *The China Study*, a comprehensive study on nutrition? Maybe we'll disagree with the conclusions, but why wouldn't we investigate? Why wouldn't we explore what we thought and decide for ourselves what is best for our bodies, genetically, generationally, and gastronomically? Why wouldn't we at least give it a try for a few weeks, days, or a month?

It's not what we do for a moment in time, (though, for some, it is); it's what we may be doing subconsciously to ourselves consistently. When we die, no one can do anything about it.

Chapter 46

The Vacation

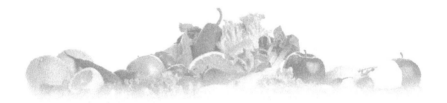

We vacationed in beautiful Sonoma County where the food and wine were so tempting and we never wanted to see the good times end. Afterward, my husband said he gained about three pounds, not as much as he normally does. I'm not sure how that happened. He's kidding me, right? Maybe he didn't have his fill during dinners and maintained a healthy portion of appetizers. Why? Was he already used to smaller portions? That would seem successful enough, right? I don't think it was because he was conscious of it, though. Was it out of habit? For my husband to be conscious enough to refrain from overindulging wouldn't even sound right. Seriously. And I know a lot of us are just as guilty—me included!

Eating only vegetables does fill you up a lot more than meat can; the professor and physician were right. As I discussed earlier, something about vegetables and grains tells our brains that we've had enough. You really should see *Forks Over Knives*. You can also find studies on YouTube on this process of how you get filled up quicker. (Did I not say how easy it is to find information?) But we have discovered that getting used to eating a lot of vegetables has trained us to eat more of them. Whether their conclusions are debatable or not, who can argue with eating more fruits and vegetables? How about more legumes? I think this diet has showed us it's okay to have another serving of asparagus or salad or, better yet, as a main entrée. Sometimes that's all we're having for dinner and, if done right, we are eating a lot of it.

Like our addictions to foods, we might have the same addictions in some sort of warped way. We might be eating more of the plant-based foods instead of the (are you ready for this?) filet mignon, cheese, and even chicken. That's right. The only way I can explain how my husband didn't gain weight is that maybe he was more inclined to eat what he was already used to. You might think, "What a concept!" Right? Either way, he was eating less . . . on vacation.

We know that controlling our portions will help us to not overeat and lose weight. Let's be real. Not until I experienced it, by learning the hard way, did this make sense. Do we change our eating habits and *then* change our minds? Or do we change our minds and *then* our eating habits? For some, changing our minds and then changing our eating habits seems to be the cause of a cycle of on-and-off weight loss. (*I need to lose weight so I'm going on a diet . . ..*) What people believe is why there are so many fad diets. We decide to lose weight, go on a diet program, and then find it hard to follow because we still believe steak is protein and cheese is necessary for our bones and miss them rightly so. Filling up faster on plant-based foods, however, truly fills us up. We have created a habit and experience that just eating smaller portions can't do it for us and especially by believing steak and cheese are good for us. When we went on vacation, this is probably what my husband already knew before going. One plateful and his brain probably told him he'd had enough. It's the only way I can make sense of it. How can you go on vacation and only gain a few extra pounds unless you didn't overeat? There is no other way.

My husband hasn't had milk in months since we began our journey too. A great talent my husband has is the ability to stick with a goal. Years ago, he made a New Year's resolution never to drink dark sodas again. Before that, he would have at least a couple of sodas a day. That was more than four years ago. As I've pieced together this experiment of a lifestyle change, I've been taking notes.

Nevertheless, I keep eating and am always at war with my weight. I didn't even bother to weigh myself before and after our trip, that's why I couldn't tell you my progress. My husband keeps records and weighs himself often while I maintain my old habits of closing my eyes and dealing with the consequences afterward.

For example, I know for sure our trip to Hawaii was disastrous for both of us this past summer, just months prior to writing this book. I didn't weigh myself before we went to Hawaii; I felt it. I look at the photos and see it too. I was definitely overweight after that trip, and weighing myself before going to the wine country this time was pointless. I suppose I've gotten too used to not weighing myself. It's too depressing. My subconscious has told me to forget about it and have a good time. The truth is, a vacation can ruin any lifestyle diet.

As I'm writing this, however, I don't feel as heavy as I normally do from returning on our vacation in the wine country. Hmmm. It's amazing what we discover when tracking this. Perhaps a plant-based diet is not only good for our health but is what can drastically keep our weight down. Once we acquire the habits of a plant-based diet will we then know how to contain ourselves? We can then become fully trained on how to keep the weight off with our eyes closed.

Chapter 47
Final Thoughts

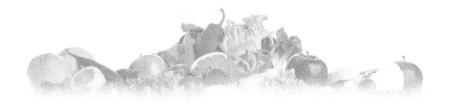

Some people believe you shouldn't announce to the world what you are trying to do before you accomplish it, but I did. I announced I was working on publishing a book about a plant-based diet to as many people as possible. I wanted to hear all the different ideas of what people thought or what interest level they had on this topic but I heard instead a lot of the same comments. Many comments came from people I knew prior to my even considering writing about this topic. I value many of those comments although I always wondered about them. All this content evidently made for great resource material. They are true stories. I didn't make up any of it. The people who will most likely recognize themselves in this book can rest assure they weren't the only ones making these comments. I don't hold anything against any of them either because I too have made the same comments. And don't our conversations with others help influence the way we think about things, including dieting?

On that note, I'm glad I let everyone know about this book. It was well received with a great amount of interest. This leads me to believe we're all confused. I had to be an investigative journalist to better understand what I was concluding because I would find a plethora of articles on the same argument. When I read how concerned some people were about bringing back cooking classes to schools, it was music to my ears. My research was often serendipitously validated!

I thought readers might be interested in knowing what happened when I adopted a plant-based diet and perhaps consider it for themselves. But, little did I know, the answers were already on the Internet and in the media. We want to know what the average person experiences before trying it. I know. I get it. I found much more information and validation for you.

I wanted to journal my first thirty days because I'm so sick and tired of hearing something is good for you one day and the next day it isn't. I don't think anyone knows for sure and it turns out there is no such thing as an absolute truth about one thing. There is a reason for the confusion. Because there are so many different types of foods and environments, it's almost impossible to conclude truth in diet. However, "when the weight of the evidence favors an idea so strongly that it can no longer be plausibly denied, we advance the ideas as a likely truth…realize that those seeking absolute proof of optimal nutrition in one or two studies will be disappointed and confused."[29]

We can all agree fruits and vegetables are good for you and the pesticides in them are bad. And with that, we have organic produce and produce with pesticides. Overall, I'm sure it's better to have Brussels sprouts filled with pesticides than a piece of steak, but competition will always exist between the blogger wanting attention and the corporation securing its sales. It's part of living in a capitalistic society.

We need to evaluate what we're eating for ourselves and stop relying on what others tell us what is good. Only you will know what is good for you by the way you feel. We should learn how to cook from a young age. Obesity is a problem because people don't know how or what to cook. We've become too

---

29   This explanation was taken from *The China Study*, in the chapter called "A House of Proteins" pg. 39.

reliant on the foods that are easy to microwave or pick up without even getting out of our cars. Or are we just too busy arguing about whose job it is to cook? And like everything else, we most likely have to treat this problem at the root of it. It's not only about eating well. We may need to go back further and promote cooking classes in middle school. Isn't this the age when some kids have to cook for themselves because their parents are at work?

One last thing: Today I picked up a catalog from our local hospital, which is considered to be one of the best in Los Angeles. It's where celebrities go, along with their paparazzi. The front page read, "Stroke incidence is rising in adults under 50. From prevention to research: How we strike back." We seem to have a surge of strokes in young people. Yes, we're no longer dealing with diabetes in younger people the way we used to, but now we're dealing with strokes. This is the first article and news I've heard about this, so I started reading. I'll get to the second article in a minute.

The lead article, titled "Unbreakable," is about a young, vibrant, athletic, twenty-eight-year-old female who suffered from a stroke. Her stroke was not about the overall condition of her health as much as it was about the defects she already had in her heart. The doctors were still researching her recovery, but this wasn't surprising. I know healthy, active people still have heart attacks, strokes, and cancer. What this article primarily talked about was the rise in strokes in people under the age of fifty-five in particular. What is scary is that the hospital or emergency room may not detect that you are having a stroke if you are young. The culprits have been found in sodas and over-the-counter dietary supplements. Laurie Paletz, a board-certified public health nurse and coordinator of the stroke program at Cedars-Sinai says, "We're seeing 24-year-olds with high cholesterol levels because they've been eating fast food for years . . . We have to get the message out to young people that strokes do happen, and the choices they make can affect their risk."[30] But here the experts go again. Dr. P. Lyden, chair of the Department of Neurology, director of the stroke program, and the Carmen and Louis Warschaw Chair in Neurology at Cedars-Sinai Hospital in Los Angeles, says, "It is important to note that not every stroke is preventable or caused by

---

30   One of the nurses who speaks up in Cedars-Sinai Winter 2015 edition of *Discoveries*.

poor health habits."[31] The young woman was relatively healthy but I think it only tells one part of the story and not its entirety. As they say, we still have a lot more research to do, you and I included.

I agree that congenital heart defects, birth control pills, and long stretches of sitting or standing contribute to blood clots, not to mention migraine headaches. The importance of informing young people about drugs is also mentioned because they also cause strokes. But it also stated that amphetamines, similar to BMPEA, an addictive ingredient found in diet products, are extremely dangerous.[32] We are consuming dietary supplements to fight weight gain, but we are unable to control, let alone understand, the side effects.

I worked with another gal who said she burned at least three hundred to four hundred calories at the gym regularly but couldn't understand why she wasn't losing weight. I was not surprised because maybe it had to do with the microwaveable mashed potatoes, corn, and turkey she ate at lunch. But who was I to tell her? I'm not an expert. Luckily for her, though, she asked a doctor and the doctor told her. She was eating way too many carbohydrates. For someone like her, how much easier would it have been to take an over-the-counter dietary supplement along with her meat protein? I've taken dietary supplements and had better workouts and I can tell you, I don't burn that many calories at the gym on any given day without something like that.

Regardless, Dr. Lyden admits, "All of this evidence seems to underscore two things: There's something to be said for moderation, and we still have much more to learn about many of the substances we ingest and the impact they have on stroke risk." I agree.

Paletz says, "Young people can take steps to reduce other risk factors. Many are the same health-conscious measures their grandparents have already

---

31   Although there is new information on increasing amounts of "over-the-counter dietary supplements, and the consumption of sodas . . . evidence is just starting to take shape and more research is needed." Quoted from Dr. Lyden in the same article.

32   Dr. Lyden says, "Amphetamine stimulants can increase blood pressure, heart rate, and body temperature; lead to serious cardiovascular complications (including stroke) at high doses; suppress sleep and appetite; and be addictive." In the U.S., the FDA has yet to recall the products or issue a public health alert. Winter 2015 edition of *Discoveries,* a Cedars-Sinai magazine.

adopted."[33] She urges young people to cut way back on sugary foods and eat a lot more fruits, vegetables, and grains. Sounds simple to me.

There is also a blueprint regarding a path to prevention that caught my attention mentioning that Alzheimer's can be managed by decreasing blood sugar levels.[34] Studies are coming out that show how higher blood sugar levels can trigger Alzheimer's but this magazine with all these articles is just something I picked up from our mail while I was in the kitchen having something to drink. I wasn't doing any research and this sure isn't a source for an extensive study, but I find any information on the latest discoveries of interest to help me better understand diet and health. I'm just telling you what I picked up.

However, I knew I would find something even more validating in the next article concerning prostate cancer. I discovered my husband would endure some serious side effects if he did not manage his bad eating habits. He would drink three to four cups of soda a day or eat a burrito with nothing but avocado and steak. It was important for him to understand this. Men are less likely to follow health advice or go to the doctor, let alone eat healthier.

For this reason, Cedars-Sinai has adopted a program called Active Surveillance for prostate cancer patients to go through. This program includes joining a men's eating and living study (known as MEAL). "The study investigates whether a plant-based diet, along with a healthy lifestyle, can help decrease progression and anxiety in men being treated with active surveillance."[35] I'm not making this up, folks! The patient who is followed in this article has lost a little weight but, more importantly, has been able to keep his prostate cancer under control.

I understand from writing this book and from reading this article that if we get hit with that dreadful C word, instead of being the victim, we can be in control. Dr. Hyung Kim, director of Academic Urology at Cedars-Sinai, says, "Instead of feeling like a victim, the patient is now in the driver's seat."[36]

---

33 A comment in the sidebar on causes and prevention of strokes in the Cedars-Sinai Winter 2015 magazine edition.

34 The blueprint I also found in the Winter 2015 issue of the magazine that is most likely a combination of recommendations by the Cedars-Sinai hospital in general.

35 A newsletter style article in the Cedars-Sinai Winter 2015 magazine regarding prostate cancer patients.

36 Dr. Kim's response just reveals how medical physicians are working towards finding ways to promote healthier eating in a separate article regarding cancer patients in the Winter 2015

I was surprised to learn that fewer than 11 percent of prostate cancer cases are fatal. I thought it was the other way around, but I also learned that "ninety percent of men diagnosed undergo some combination of surgery, radiation, and hormone therapy, which is often unnecessary and can result in serious side effects that noticeably diminish (their) quality of life."[37] The Active Surveillance program helps patients enroll in a study where a plant-based diet can be monitored. What is not surprising is that many hospitals and doctors are unwilling to follow this regimen or at least study it. The article closes out with saying that the patient being followed "eats lots of leafy greens, consumes very little red meat, and drinks alcohol in moderation." I asked myself, "Why not get my husband on this plant-based diet now?"

It's everywhere. Everything we want to know about living healthier is in front of us more than ever. For me, it landed on my kitchen counter in the form of a local hospital magazine. While I sip my tea and read the magazine lying on my kitchen counter, I am without excuses.

I was stunned and sort of excited about this book. Talking to people about my book got the conversations going and, from this, I gained feedback on how people think about what they eat. Some people are dead set on having their meat and dairy even though there is a mix of doctors that promote these foods and some that don't but all promote fruits and vegetables and to eat a lot of them.

Without sounding too harsh, I want to relay what I observed. I heard the same questions and answers from a lot of people. Do we all have the same beliefs about food? If we do, these beliefs and opinions were originated from somewhere. In the previously mentioned book by Chase Chandler, *The Wealthy Family*, I was surprised to find a quote by Vladimir Lenin. It's a quote we may find true, even from someone with such opposing beliefs to our country: "A lie told often enough becomes the truth."[38]

A whole food, plant-based diet is not really a diet. It's rather a description of the kinds of foods I'm eating. It's not a diet I'm trying to lose weight on, it's a diet I'm trying to be more educated for optimal health reasons. I need to

---

magazine.

37   The same article on prostate cancer patients written by Jasmine Aimaq.

38   Even though we may have been educated on how to eat by the meat and dairy industries for so long, do we begin to believe it as truth?

learn more about it, which means I need to learn how to cook using plant-based foods. Eating more fruits and vegetables is hard because I don't think we know how to eat more fruits and vegetables. We don't know how to cook or what to think about what is good and what isn't. We're political about healthcare and adamant about eating the very foods that aren't good for us. Our refrigerator was filled with the foods that, at the very least, should be eaten in moderation and not every week. The answers are right in front of us, but we don't want to accept them. A friend said that when she sat down to eat, she had to feel as if she were having a meal because salads were not as filling for her. Did she mean not as *fulfilling*?

I'm not the authority on what is good for you and I'm still learning. It's clear to me, though, and even Richard too. I succumbed to heating up a bowl of carnitas and beans when Richard asked why we were having meat, let alone a frozen dinner. A bell went off. James Allen, in his book *As a Man Thinketh*, a classic in personal development, writes, "Change of diet will not help a man who will not change his thoughts. When a man makes his thoughts pure, he no longer desires impure food."[39] I thought having a quick and easy meal to pull out of the freezer was a convenience. But his comment led me to believe my thoughts were still not aligned with my beliefs and evidently were not helping my body become healthy as I intended.

What if young kids were taught how to cook vegetables in many different ways? What if harmful substances were removed from the store shelves? What if hospitals promoted plant-based diets more? (Or do they already and we're not listening?) Stephen Freedland, MD at Cedars-Sinai Hospital, says, "Health advice often falls on deaf ears until a disease with a scary name makes an appearance."[40]

I'm not sure what would happen, but I don't want any of those things to happen. Richard and I have changed our minds on what we are eating and we are exercising more. We are reversing the psychology of bad eating habits and filling ourselves up faster. It's a quest to no longer want what's not good for us.

---

39 The context for this quote is written to describe how pure thoughts build up a body's strength. With pure thoughts, the body will respond like the thoughts of one's diet. This quote can be found on page 34.

40 This was a side note reference to the article regarding prostate cancer in the Winter 2015 edition of *Discoveries*, the Cedars-Sinai Medical Hospital quarterly magazine.

We are not 100 percent vegan, plant-based, vegetarian, or anything like that. We have simply learned how to transform our eating habits that are *slowly* becoming more plant-based. We accept our failures, keep trying, keep learning, and realize that what we eat is a lifelong process but, most importantly, our responsibility.

What are your challenges?

Chapter 48

Favorite Plant-Based Recipes

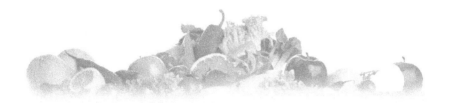

Here are my favorite recipes (made for two servings) that I talk about throughout the book. Read how I prepared them, but feel free to create your own by researching different ways to make these dishes. Pick up a plant-based cookbook or just go on Google like I did and if the recipes look easy enough to follow, try them. This is how I was able to learn more about dishes I could make without meat and butter and create a much lighter dish. In no time, I have created favorite ways to make these dishes sometimes with ingredients I had in my cupboards for years. These recipes I share have been just a blueprint to help us transition into healthier eating.

And, yes, they are all in the right category. I've learned to have what would normally be an appetizer for dinner and find it just as filling. That's one of the reasons I categorized everything. It's liberating not to have the same customs I grew up with that were making me fat. Have fun!

BREAKFAST

Pineapple, Peanut Butter, and Almond Milk Smoothie

I buy pineapple often and know how to cut one in about 2 minutes. I grab the biggest, heaviest knife I have, cut the top off, and then the sides holding it up—the only big fruit I cut properly. The bottom is a cinch to cut off and the rest is easy until Richard pointed out that he didn't eat the center. I had forgotten about that. I think we don't eat enough of this delicious fruit fresh because we don't know how to pick a good one nor do we know how long to leave it on the counter before cutting it. Do we figure it's too cumbersome to cut? Dole has made a killing off canned pineapple (as well as pineapples). I was at the grocery store when I was picking one up and an older gentleman asked me how to know if it was ripe enough. I can't remember who told me (probably my mom), but if you can pick the very top of the leaf easily, it's ready.

When I cut pineapple and store it in a plastic container in the fridge, it hardly lasts; we love it so much. However, a good smoothie to try is a pineapple and peanut butter smoothie.

½ cup fresh pineapple (with no center)
2 cubes of ice (or crushed ice)
2 tablespoons of peanut butter
1 cup of vanilla or plain plant milk
Blend all in a blender and enjoy!

Tarzan Smoothie

I'm learning how to drink this smoothie although my mom is already a pro at it. I don't know why I think I'm drinking a jungle, but it's one of those paradigms that make me think I'm drinking a bitter jungle when, in reality, it's not bad at all. It's actually very refreshing. Here goes nothing.

½ cup of spinach
¼ cucumber with skin removed
½ of a celery stalk

Juice of 1 lime

½ cup of coconut water (pulp is okay)

2 ice cubes or crushed ice

Blend all in a blender and enjoy!

Gluten-free Cocoa Muffins

If you ever see these, grab them! Cocoa has been on my grocery list, although I'm not much of a baker. However, I have hardly had a bad gluten free chocolate muffin. Udis has some gluten-free chocolate muffins that are worth their price, but if you're a baker, make these. Replace the butter with applesauce, use coconut flower instead of white flour, and add chocolate chips or even nuts if you like that kind of stuff. Richard went looking for them in the fridge when I bought them and I think he was upset I ate the last one.

Potato Pancakes

I've always loved these and now I like them more. I typically only make them when there are leftover mashed potatoes (for heavens sake, don't make mashed potatoes just for these) and they are pretty satisfying. You can order them with cheese, bacon, and egg but you really don't need all that. Trust me.

Leftover mashed potatoes

Egg white or egg replacer

Chives

Salt and pepper

Coconut oil

Gluten-free flower

Arugula, sprouts, or other greens

Mushrooms if desired

Heat a skillet or non-stick pan on medium heat. Take the leftover mashed potatoes and stir in chives and salt and pepper to taste. Make balls out of them at whatever size you choose. Flatten and brush with egg replacer and then coat them with flower. Pour coconut oil into the pan and place pancakes into the pan.

Heat for about 2-3 minutes each side. Remove from heat and add arugula or other greens on top and serve. Can be served with grilled tomatoes, mushrooms and avocado if desired.

Sweet Potato Pancakes

Sweet potatoes to the rescue! I have replaced adding all the milk and eggs in the pancake batter when it calls for it. I like the pancake batter where all you have to do is add water, but if you have a pancake mix that calls for oil and eggs, this will work.

> 1 sweet potato or yam, cooked and squashed
> ½ recommended serving of gluten-free pancake mix (Use whatever pancake mix—as long as it doesn't have white bleached flower added to it.)
> Your favorite plant milk (If needed according to mix.)
> Eggs or egg replacer, although the sweet potatoes mixed with plant milk should be enough as a binding agent. I use egg replacer equivalent to 1 egg and it works fine. I just make sure the egg replacer is now mixed more on the thin side than thick if I'm using it.
> 1 tablespoon ground flax seed
> 1 tablespoon vanilla-flavored shake mix (Use your favorite—plant-based is better, but whatever you like is best to use.)
> ½ teaspoon of coconut oil per pancake

Try to avoid the vegetable oil where possible or just use half of what is recommended.

Heat the griddle. Blend everything together according to pancake mix, including the smashed sweet potato, flax seed, and shake mix.[41] If making pancake mix from scratch, Google homemade pancakes, crepes, waffles, or whatever you're making and replace the flower with half of the large, cooked sweet potato. Use plant milk and egg replacer as suggested. Mix the batter with the sweet potato until it has a good consistency. Spread a ½ teaspoon of coconut oil on the griddle

---

41   I understand not everyone will agree with the shake mix addition because they tend to have a lot of additives but I allow for everyone to make their own way. What's important is to learn how to get creative with everyday foods.

for each pancake and pour the batter onto the griddle. Instead of butter, use ½ teaspoon of coconut oil for pancakes if desired and serve with fruit.[42]

Dairy-free, Gluten-free French Toast

How do I do this, you ask? I find every bit of substitution I can find but I found this recipe online and tweaked it a bit. Richard loved them! Miracles do happen.

Your favorite gluten-free bread (Mine is Udis raisin bread but their plain bread is good too.)

Egg replacer
1 ½ cup of plant milk (Vanilla and/or coconut almond milk is good.)
1 teaspoon of vanilla
1 tablespoon of ground flax seed (if desired)
1 tablespoon coconut oil (if desired)
Pancake syrup

Heat your skillet on high. Make the equivalent of 2 eggs with egg replacer and mix with all the rest of the ingredients. Add half of the coconut oil to the skillet or pan. Dip your bread in the mixture and set on skillet or pan. Cook for about 4 minutes on each side or longer than you're used to. (I think the egg replacer takes longer to cook.) When you remove them from the skillet, coat slightly with other half of coconut oil if desired. Serve immediately with fresh berries and warm syrup.

Sweet Potatoes Period

I saw this online and thought how brilliant it was. It's so easy too and I think it was a way to get the kids to eat sweet potatoes—in my case, it was my husband.

1 baked sweet potato, peeled and cubed
Pancake syrup
Pecans if desired

---

42 Other plant foods to use besides sweet potatoes are bananas, applesauce, squashed blueberries, or raspberries, etc. The idea is whatever you can get squishy.

With a fork, pierce the sweet potato a few times and set in microwave for about 4-5 minutes on high. Gently, peel the skin and cut the warm sweet potatoes in cubes. Put on a cute dish and drizzle syrup on them. How can anyone resist breakfast with syrup on a cute dish?

LUNCH

Potato Tacos
    2 potatoes, peeled and cut into cubes
    Herbs such as rosemary, thyme, or marjoram or your favorite spice
    Olive oil
    Avocado
    2 tomatoes, diced
    4 corn tortillas
    Homemade Pico de Gallo[43]
    Cilantro, arugula, or chopped mixed salad to garnish

Turn on oven to about 375°. Peel and cut potatoes into cubes. Boil potatoes for about 10 minutes being careful not to overcook them. Keep checking them with a fork and if you can easily pierce them, they are done. Take out a cookie sheet and oil the pan. Dice tomatoes and avocado. Remove and strain potatoes. Put them in a bowl and toss with a spatula in olive oil. Season with favorite seasonings or herbs and set aside to cool for about another 10 minutes before putting them on the cookie sheet. Put them in the oven to bake or for faster results, put them in the broiler for about 3 minutes. Keep a close eye on them if they are put in the broiler. I like to put mine in my mini toaster oven just long enough to brown.

Heat tortillas on a skillet on both sides. When potatoes are done, put avocado, potatoes, tomato, and homemade salsa in that order in a warm tortilla. Garnish with cilantro or arugula if desired.

---

43   Recipe is coming up ahead if you don't know how to make it.

Lentil Soup

I make all kinds of lentil soup even though I grew up on the dark brown lentil soup with cilantro. My favorite lentils are the red lentils. They look like barley and have this healthy look in my soup but its just lentils. This has been the soup I prepare often that I can make in a small saucepan in about 10 minutes for lunch. When done right, its colorful and beautiful. It's Pinterest quality.

¼ cup or ¼ bag of red lentils

1 Roma tomato, chopped

3 garlic cloves

1 large carrot cut julienne style

½ corn on the cob

1 cup cabbage of any kind except purple (It can turn the water purple.)

Vegan or gluten-free cube of vegetable bouillon

¼ bunch of cilantro

4 cups water

Add water to a medium size saucepan and turn on heat to high. Add the lentils. Smash the garlic cloves and put those in the water with the bouillon. Cut the carrots and add those in the saucepan. Chop the tomato and cabbage. When the soup is boiling, add the tomato and cabbage and lower the heat to medium. Add ½ (or 1 corn on the cob cut in two for two people) in the pot. When the water starts to simmer again, add the cilantro. Heat for another 2 minutes and serve immediately.

SIDE GARNISHES AND SPREADS

Homemade Pico de Gallo

I'm including jalapenos as a staple in my fridge just to always be able to make this in a pinch. It's such a great addition to tacos, soups, or vegetables that I never thought of to always have in the fridge. Jalapenos add a great spicy heat that is so good for us too. I always thought to pick up salsa but this has turned out to be a better choice, although Richard still buys salsa in a jar all the time.

2 tomatoes diced very small (use pairing knife for best results)

½ onion diced very small (use onion slicer and then go back and dice for best results)

1 jalapeno (make sure to remove the stem, vine, and seeds with the same pairing knife or you will die from the heat)

½ a bunch of chopped cilantro (chop half the bunch from the side, not across the top, fold, and chop as fine as you can get it)

½ a lemon or lime

Dice everything and put into bowl. Squeeze half a lemon over it and toss. Voila!

Corn Salsa

Everyone knows this one. I saw this and made up my own but it's very similar to the typical corn salsa on the Internet. Nonetheless, I would recommend making a big bowl when doing this because, as most of you know who have made this dish, it goes quick—especially at a gathering.

3 fresh corns (frozen bag of corn works good too)

2 cups of cooked black beans, drained

1 large onion, diced

3 Roma tomatoes, diced

2 jalapenos, diced

1 bunch of cilantro

1 lime

Cook the corn on the cobs for about 10 minutes—until it boils. Remove the corn and set aside to cool. Drain the cooked black beans and put in a large bowl. Add the onion, tomato, jalapeno, and cilantro. When the corns have cooled, remove the corn from their cobs with a corn cutter. Put all the corn in the bowl with the rest of the mixture. Squeeze all the juice from the lime right into the mixture and fold everything gently with a spatula. Season with salt, pepper, or use Tajin seasoning to your desired taste. Salsa can be chilled and ready to eat later or served right away. It's great with corn chips and guacamole.

Garlic Spread with Orange, Lemon, and Ginger

I found this at that farmer's market and I swear I'm going to keep making it to get it the way I want. I will never forget a first love. A way to get a good spread going with garlic is to roast the garlic. I cut the ends of the cloves and, with the skin still on, I put them in my toaster for about 6-8 minutes. If they're not cooked thoroughly and aren't mushy enough, I put them in for another few minutes. (I have done this and refrigerated them to prepare later and it lasts a long time.) I even heard Carmen Diaz talk about grilling shallots as a spread in her book and storing it in her fridge too.

2 garlic cloves
1 tablespoon of orange juice
½ teaspoon of orange zest
1 tablespoon of lemon juice
½ teaspoon of lemon zest
½ teaspoon of ginger zest

Grind roasted garlic in a mortar and pestle, adding the juices and then the zests. Add the ginger last and taste. Add more juice for consistency and zest for stronger flavors. Serve with crackers, cucumbers, raw tomatoes, and roasted vegetables or on toast. Go for it!

Beet Spread

I love beets but I know a lot of people don't. What's worse is beets go remarkably well with goat cheese and a lot of people don't like goat cheese either. Although I'm eating a lot less cheese these days, premade beets processed with goat cheese is like a dream. However, I prepared this as a transitional dish. I found a vegan beet spread recipe online that I pinned on my plant-based Pinterest board to try later but I'm going to give you what I made during my first 26 days.

1 jar of premade beets,[44] diced
2 ounces of goat cheese, diced
1 tablespoon of diced tarragon
½ teaspoon of coarse sea salt
1 teaspoon of extra-virgin olive oil

Dice and then blend everything gently in a bowl with a spatula and serve over sliced cucumbers on rice crackers. People will think you have such an advanced palate.

Raw Organic Almonds
If you see these, try them. I was surprised by how flavorful these were. If you see the most pure kind, try them. They're a little more expensive but if you can find them by the pound, buy them.

Pistachios
This is the most under-valued nut there is. It's great for desserts, snacks, home made nut mixes, and baking. I like these on top of ice cream but I have to watch the fat content.

APPETIZERS

Roasted Corn with Garlic Spread and Chili Lime Spice
Nothing compares to buttered corn except a vegan spread and Tajin lime spice. Once you have a solid spread like the roasted garlic spread made with maybe just lemon this time, you can use that instead of butter and, guess what? It will be more flavorful and you may never go back to bland margarine again.

2 corns
1 Head of Garlic
½ Lemon juice

---

44 Beets can also be baked for about an hour—that is the better choice.

Grill or boil corn. Broil or roast the garlic peeled or unpeeled. If roasting unpeeled, the skin will come off but you have to remove them quickly to peel and put back in the broiler. When done, place garlic in mortar and pestle and grind. Add lemon juice salt and use to smother corn. Put corn back on the grill and heat a little more. Add a little salt if desired.

Marinated Mushrooms

I made these and they were delicious. This is a great appetizer to change things up. This is from my library of recipes. When I make up something that actually tastes good, I record it. It's just another way to journal. Good thing I had this to share. I don't remember where I got this or how I was inspired to make it, but here it goes.

½ cup extra-virgin olive oil
2 pounds of cremini or button mushrooms
2 lemons, juiced with about 1 tablespoon of zest
3 garlic cloves, sliced
1 small bunch of fresh thyme
2 bay leaves
Salt and fresh ground pepper

Add ¼ cup of olive oil to large skillet over medium heat. Add mushrooms and cook for about 3 minutes. Remove from heat and stir in lemon zest and juice, garlic, thyme, and bay leaves. Pour remaining olive oil and season mixture with salt and pepper. Pour into bowl and allow to cool. Serve at room temperature over crackers, cucumbers or with toothpicks.

Lentil Salad

I've seen this salad and I'm still thinking about which kind of lentils I would use. I'm not too crazy about the brown lentils, but there's also a French green kind I should look for. I like the rustic look of them. Lentils are good in soup because, otherwise, their texture sticks to your teeth. I can't describe it any other way, which is why I'm not sure how people could eat them without them swimming in water. However, a good way to make this salad is with a lot of vegetables like celery, onion, persimmon, and maybe even cucumber. Get creative.

Salad with Homemade Dressing

There are hundreds of ways to make salads. We all know this but the best way to make a salad is to prepare your own homemade salad dressing. Richard is still having a hard time with homemade dressing, but one way I won him over was with a recipe from *Food52 Genius Recipes*[45] with roasted carrots that he insists we prepare when we have company over. It is that good. In the same spirit of sharing a remarkable dish, I'll share with you the homemade dressing that inspired even my picky husband, thanks to ABC Kitchen restaurant in New York City. Perhaps it was the roasted orange and lemon? Here's the dressing:

1 orange, one half juiced, the other left whole

1 lemon, one half juiced, the other left whole

½ cup extra-virgin olive oil

1 teaspoon cumin seeds (Although I think I just used ground cumin which is what I had.)

2 medium garlic cloves

1 tablespoon fresh thyme leaves

1 teaspoon red wine vinegar

1 teaspoon crushed red pepper flakes

Fresh ground black pepper

1 tablespoon sugar

Combine 1 teaspoon each of the orange and lemon juices, 2 tablespoons of olive oil, the cumin, garlic, thyme, vinegar, and red pepper flakes in a blender and blend until smooth. Season the marinade to taste with salt and pepper then squeeze the juice from the roasted citrus halves into a small bowl. Add remaining fresh citrus juices, remaining 6 tablespoons of olive oil, and the

---

45   If you haven't discovered *Food52 Genius Recipes*, you should. Although there are a lot of meat dishes, these recipes are rustic and creatively made in ways that *train* us how to cook differently. Check out *Food52 Genius Recipes*, a book I've cherished that was a true gift from a dear friend.

sugar. Season the dressing to taste with salt and pepper and whisk to combine. This dressing was added to the roasted carrots called *Roasted Carrot & Avocado Salad with Crunchy Seeds.*[46]

Spinach Salad with Strawberries, Walnuts, Chia Seeds, and Balsamic Vinaigrette

I love this salad. Adding strawberries to spinach salad makes the squeaky fresh spinach that sticks to your teeth more bearable. Use this salad with a citrus or champagne dressing and it will be hard not to get anyone to eat their spinach. Sunflower seeds are a nice touch too. I think I'll make this tonight!

Cauliflower Soup

This is the second part of the cauliflower steak recipe from *Food52 Genius Recipes* but this soup can stand on its own. I'd also like to share a nice touch I just learned. The other night, we went to a plant-based restaurant and they made this beautiful cauliflower consume that was delicious. When you make this soup, add a dash of walnut or spicy oil on top with pine nuts or any other of your favorite nuts as a garnish. It was divine!

1 head of cauliflower
Salt and pepper
2 garlic cloves
1 cup of water
¾ cup plain plant milk
Parsley for garnish

Here, you want to boil the cauliflower and garlic in the water and plain plant milk for around 8-10 minutes. When they're nice and tender, remove the cauliflower but reserve the liquid. Transfer the cauliflower to a blender and add about ½ cup of the remaining liquid. Puree until smooth and add more of the liquid to find the consistency you want. Return the puree to the same saucepan that you boiled the cauliflower in and dispose the rest of the liquid. Heat again

---

46   *Food52 Genius Recipes* by Kristen Miglore. Ten-Speed Press, pages 82-83.

and serve immediately. Garnish with a spicy oil such as a red pepper oil, chopped nuts, and parsley (for color).

Butternut Squash Soup

I was just talking to my mom about this. I love butternut squash (or any winter squash) soup, cauliflower soup, tomato soup, split pea soup, potato soup—you name it. If it gets squishy, let me put it in the blender to make a nice puree. These soups only take a few ingredients too, which is nice. I still explore the Internet for different recipes, but here is the gist of a good winter squash soup.

> 1 butternut squash, cut into cubes and steamed—boiled in about 1 cup of water in a large pot.
> 1 large chopped carrot (about ½ cup)
> ½ medium sweet (white) onion, chopped
> 1 cup water or plant milk
> 1 cup vegetable broth[47]
> ½ teaspoon of coarse sea salt

Put about 1 cup of water in a large pot and add the butternut squash cubes and chopped carrot and put on medium heat for about 20 minutes. Add water if the pot looks like it's burning, trying not to submerge in water but just enough to cook. Heat a non-stick frying pan until it's hot. Add the sweet onion and stir for about a minute and, just before it starts to stick, add the vegetable broth. Let the onions cook until they're transparent and the broth has been soaked up a bit. Remove the steamy squash and carrot, making sure they are cooked through from the other big pot and put portions in a blender. (You may have to do this in batches). Add half of the water or plant milk and the onion mixture. Puree and put back in a saucepan to heat by adding salt to taste. Serve immediately. These

---

47 You can rely on buying the organic kind or just make vegetable broth yourself. I found a round basket with a chain that I could use to boil vegetables (that I know will go bad if I don't eat them in the next day or so) with garlic and onion. I chop everything and place it in the basket and boil in water. I take that water and store it in a large glass container and use on whatever needs vegetable broth.

soups don't taste as good frozen but can be put in the fridge for later. I would cut everything and store to easily take out to cook. It's perfect when just made.

DINNER

Ratatouille—look online for this delicious recipe. I have made this but it didn't come out the way I wanted. However, it's one of those dishes I'll most likely try again *because* it looks so beautiful.

Bean Chili

This is probably one of the most popular "vegan" dishes there is. There are hundreds of recipes online for this and it's one of those dishes that can replace a meat-eater's temptation. There are so many, like black beans, pinto beans, white beans, red beans—you name it. When cooked with tomatoes, onion, and even carrots, you have yourself a meal. I only made this once and used beer. I found the recipe in my library of recipes that happen to be among the delicious ribs, meatloaf, pork chops, and halibut recipes. For the sake of this book, I'll show you my chili recipe but I'm removing the bacon and ground turkey. It's good, but you'll mostly have to work on your palate if you miss the meat.

> 1 onion
> 2 cups of cooked beans, strained
> 1 teaspoon of cumin
> ½ bottle of beer
> 1/3 bag of frozen corn
> 1 bunch of cilantro chopped
> 1 avocado
> Corn tortillas
> 1 tomato, diced
> 1 teaspoon of onion powder
> 1 teaspoon of garlic powder
> 2 tablespoons of your favorite hot sauce (Mine is called "Valentina.")
> 1 tablespoon of olive oil

Fry onion in a little olive oil in a skillet for a few minutes until it starts to turn a nice brown color. Deglaze with beer, adding slowly. Add strained, cooked beans and cook for another 2 minutes. Add onion and garlic powders and cumin and stir. Add diced tomato and frozen corn and bring to a boil. When it starts to boil, turn the heat down, add your favorite hot sauce, and mix it up. Let it cool for a few minutes and serve warm. Garnish with cilantro and/or avocado and serve with warm corn tortillas.

Nine-bean Soup

If you know how to make soup, you know how to make a nice nine-bean soup. Follow instructions on the package of beans so you cook them right but make sure to add the vegetables in an order where some have to cook longer than others. For example, you want to add the carrots first because they'll take the longest to cook and tomato and herbs last because you don't want to overcook them. Remember that tomatoes make a nice tomato broth but you can always add tomato paste that you can make from scratch for a true tomato soup base. And don't ever forget the garlic. Without garlic, you'll have a soup that is very bland, unless you're into that.

Eggplant Sans Parmesan

I made this without cheese and it was incredible. I was thrilled I got a thumbs-up but if I'm having people over or it's a Sunday dinner, I'll add a little mozzarella. The key is to add only a little.

1 eggplant, skin removed and sliced
3 big garlic cloves
Tomato sauce[48]
2 tablespoons of olive oil
Fresh chopped parsley

---

48 Try making your own tomato sauce. All tomato sauces are typically in a can, which come with a lot of preservatives. It's a staple that, once you get good at it, will let you live like an Italian!

Heat a skillet. Skin the eggplant—just remove the skin. I've tried this a number of ways and I just can't seem to get the skin cooked enough to like it. Maybe it will work for you but I just haven't figured it out. Slice the eggplant sideways and pour the oil in the skillet. Place the eggplant in the skillet with the garlic and sauté for about 2-3 minutes on each side. Pour the tomato sauce over the eggplant and let it simmer for about 10 minutes. Dust with parsley flakes and season with salt and pepper to taste. Serve over your favorite pasta or let it cook for about 3-4 minutes before putting into the oven to bake with a little mozzarella on top.

Portabella Mushroom Spaghetti
I just made this dish last night but with tomato sauce and brown rice gluten-free penne pasta. Darn! It wasn't as good as this.

1 bag of spinach (green) spaghetti (We use only ½ box or bag but use whatever you're used to.)

½ bag of spinach
3 large shallots
4 big garlic cloves
2 medium-sized Portabella mushrooms
¼ cup of chopped basil
1 tablespoon of sherry
3 tablespoons of olive oil

Boil spaghetti with salt. Sauté garlic, shallots, and mushrooms in olive oil for about 2 minutes until onion caramelizes and mushrooms shrink. Add sherry and basil and continue turning in pan. Remove mushrooms and place in big serving bowl. In same pan, add more olive oil and spinach. Sauté for about 2 minutes. Drain spaghetti and pour over mushrooms. Add spinach, toss, and serve. We garnished with Cotija cheese, but I would simply garnish with fresh herbs this time. My recipe card says, "Serve with red wine." Really? Okay!

Portabella Mushroom Tacos[49]

I learned how to make these tacos from an old watering hole from my single days. The first time I had these, I couldn't believe they were vegetarian. They were delicious with a beer. They're as simple to make as the potato tacos I often eat for lunch except I use the following:

1 Portabella or 8 cremini mushrooms, sliced
1 whole onion or 3 big shallots, finely chopped
¼ cup of white wine
2 tablespoons of olive oil
Chopped flat-leaf parsley
Finely chopped salad greens for garnish
4 corn tortillas

In a heated skillet, add the oil, onions, and mushrooms. Sauté until the onions become a little browned and the mushrooms have reduced to a wilted form. Add the white wine, toss it around until the wine is reduced, and then sprinkle with the finely chopped parsley. Heat the tortillas over a skillet and pour the mushrooms and onions in each tortilla. Garnish with chopped salad, avocado, and tomato if desired.

Plant-Based Taco Supreme

I've talked about potato tacos and mushroom tacos but this would be the plant-based taco supreme. I can only eat two of these outrageously delicious tacos but it's one of the best and probably the first you should serve to help others in your household help you transition to a healthier diet. Trust me, this will be the best 10 minutes you'll have eating something healthy.

2 medium-sized russet potatoes
½ bag of cleaned and rinsed spinach

---

49 I throw anything I can find in these tacos but this is the basic way I make them. I'll add tomatoes, grilled artichoke, guacamole, and even white rice if I have some. It's hard not to have a mushroom taco with the saltiness of the crumbled cheese, which I'm still trying to find an alternative for. Cotija cheese is great on this taco.

½ bunch of cilantro, chopped

1 whole tub of Cremini mushrooms, sliced

½ onion

4 tablespoons of coconut oil

1 tablespoon of olive oil

4 regular size corn tortillas

Turn on oven at 375°. Bring a pot of water to a boil. Skin and cube the potatoes and add the potatoes to the pot, being careful not to splash boiling water on yourself. Boil until potatoes are cooked through. Drain potatoes and season with salt, pepper, or other spicy seasoning and mix with olive oil using a spatula, being careful not to break up the potatoes. Place potatoes on a cookie sheet and bake for about 20 minutes. Heat a skillet or non-stick pan on high until it's hot. Add coconut oil, onion, and mushrooms and sauté for about 2 minutes. Add spinach and sauté until cooked through. Take potatoes out of oven and let cool for about 5 minutes. Put potatoes in corn tortilla and top with spinach and mushrooms. Garnish with chopped cilantro.

Curry Potatoes

I've made curry potatoes a few times because it's just delicious. An item I like to keep on hand is coconut milk. The light milk doesn't work as well as the heavier coconut milk but I just can't believe I've had curry in my cupboards for years and never used it. Now I cook with it all the time to make with potatoes.

2 medium potatoes cubed

3 large carrots

½ of a cauliflower (if desired)

1 frozen bag of peas

1 tablespoon of curry powder

1 can of coconut milk

5 tablespoons of olive oil

1 onion, chopped or thinly sliced

1 tablespoon of ground cumin

1 teaspoon of ground turmeric

1 tablespoon of ground coriander

½ teaspoon of salt

"In a large, heavy-bottomed skillet, heat the oil over medium heat. When hot, add the hot curry powder and stir it around for 30 seconds. Add the onions to the pan and sauté until they are tender and a bit golden. Add the carrots, potatoes, and minced garlic. Give it all a good stir, and then add about a half-cup each of water and coconut milk. Stir in the turmeric, salt, and coriander. Reduce the heat to low and cover it. Check every so often to stir the pot and check the moisture level. When the moisture is almost all absorbed, add more coconut milk and water, in equal parts. Continue to cook, stir, and add liquid until the vegetables are very tender and the curry is nice and thick. At this point, taste it to check that the spice levels are where you like them. When you're there, stir in the peas and the rest of the coconut milk (and water if necessary), and cook it for another 3 minutes or so, until the peas are heated through and the curry thickens up again. Serve over brown rice. Makes 4 generous servings."[50]

Easy Stir-fry

If you don't have a wok, now would be a good time to get one. A wok becomes your best friend other than a food processor if you want to eat healthy foods. Make sure to get a wooden flat spoon too, as it works well with the wok.

¼ pound of snow peas

1 bag of fresh sprouts

3 large carrots cut julienne style (I don't like the already cut carrots in a bag—they come out squishy for some reason unless they're finely chopped. Just peel and cut them.)

4-5 big cloves of garlic

---

50 This was the best explanation of how I do it. Not surprising, because I learned this recipe from the Internet. This comes from http://www.thespicehouse.com/recipes/potato-curry-with-peas-and-carrots.

1 Half a package of firm tofu—unless you like a lot of it. (Tofu gets bad in the fridge quickly, so use the whole amount if you don't think you'll use the rest in the next few days.)

Sesame oil or Thai basil oil

1 teaspoon of fish sauce (Omit if you're avoiding all animal products.)

1 tablespoon of organic Tamari sauce

½ teaspoon of Chinese five-spice seasoning

Chinese chili sauce

1 cup of cooked brown rice (if not using tofu)[51]

Mix the fish sauce, Tamari, and Chinese five-spice seasoning together (and chili sauce if you have some) and set aside. Heat the wok. (Mine heats up quickly.) Pour the seasoned oil from the top all the way around until the oil gathers at the bottom. Add the carrots and garlic and stir around for about 5 minutes. Add the snow peas and fresh sprouts and toss some more for another 3 minutes. Add the tofu and brown rice or either of the two. When everything looks cooked, pour the sauce over everything and heat the sauce with the stir-fry until cooked through. Serve in a small bowl with chopped cilantro, lime, peanuts, and/or sesame seeds on top.

Pad Thai with Tofu

I grew my sphere of Italian gluten-free pastas with Asian noodles. I've been experimenting with them ever since. My favorite is Pad Thai and Richard really likes it too. Every time I make it, he says its "restaurant quality," which cracks me up. There are tons of ways to make the sauce from scratch but I typically buy a sauce that has very low sodium and additives in a jar. This is how I make it with sauce I store in my cupboards. If you want to make it from scratch, knock yourself out. You'd be amazed at how much better it probably tastes from scratch anyway. This dish is prepared very similarly to stir-fry.

1 bag of Pad Thai noodles

Half a carton of tofu, sliced and diced in cubes

---

51 If you like tofu and rice together, that's not a bad combination if you're really hungry.

1 bag of sprouts

2 large carrots, cut julienne style and very thin

1 red bell pepper, sliced and diced

½ onion

1 jalapeno or Thai pepper for a spicier taste

½ cilantro bunch, chopped

¼ cup of chopped peanuts

Pad Thai sauce

Sesame, basil, or lemongrass oil

Put a big pot of water on the stove to boil. After chopping all the vegetables, take out your wok and, just like stir-fry, heat the wok until it's really hot. Pour the oil of your choice around the top of the wok and let it slide down to the center. Add the carrots, garlic, and onion and toss for about 2 minutes. Add the bell peppers and sprouts and toss for another minute. When the water boils in the big pot, add the noodles in the boiling water and let them cook for about 2-3 minutes (instructions are right on the package). While keeping an eye on the vegetables, drain noodles, rinse, and toss right into the wok with the vegetables. Pour the sauce and blend thoroughly in the wok. Serve and garnish with cilantro, chopped peanuts, lime wedges and sliced peppers for added spice.

Newly-discovered Plant-based Tacos
Cauliflower can be made a number of ways but steamed with a chili lime spice is good for tacos. Steam the cauliflower and sauté with your favorite spices. Heat a corn tortilla and add avocado, salad and tomatoes or any other favorite vegetable. These are also a great snack when you steam cauliflowers for later and store them in the fridge for a quick snack.

Cauliflower Steaks
This is another recipe I got from *Food52 Genius Recipes*. After eating this dish as a main entrée, I read the recipe again to prepare it one more time and later read

that it was a good first course dish or appetizer. I don't care. I make this as a main dish but, instead of putting them on top of pureed cauliflower, I created a lima bean garlic puree that I learned from a lady I worked with. Hers came out more thick than mine, but I'll keep tweaking mine.

Turn the oven on at 350°. Cut the cauliflower from the center to create 2 steaks along the stem. Set aside, put the rest of the cauliflower pieces in the refrigerator for later, or brush with olive oil, salt, and cracked pepper. Heat a cast iron skillet or pan that you can transfer into the oven. You should be able to fit both steaks in a skillet. Sauté both sides for about 2-3 minutes or when nice and golden brown. After turning them over, put them both in the oven straight from the pan for about 10 minutes. Lay on top of a pureed vegetable with a side of kale salad.

Updated Zucchini Squash

This has been a favorite of mine growing up, but with a lot of cheese on top. I credit my mom for doing whatever she could to get us to eat our vegetables. Unfortunately, I hardly eat cheese anymore but this side dish is just as good without the cheese. Thanks, Mom!

2 big zucchinis, chopped or cut julienne style
½ of a medium-sized onion, chopped
1 tomato
4 garlic cloves
Fresh herbs like thyme or basil

Chop zucchini and put in sauté pan with onions and garlic. Cook for about a good minute and add tomatoes. Cover for about 5 minutes and add fresh herbs on top. Serve immediately and let your guests or family add their own salt. The fresh herbs do the trick for flavoring but everyone's palate is different. Add quinoa and you're on to something. Add tomato sauce and pour over polenta and you've got yourself a meal!

SIDE DISHES

Mashed Potatoes with Garlic Even a Farmer Would Love
Although an old favorite with butter, the butter can be replaced with garlic and the milk can be replaced with plain plant milk. The goal is the consistency and taste and both can be achieved by replacing the dairy very easily. Add a little pepper and use a ricer and you're good to go! You will impress even those from the Midwest.

Lime Rice with Cilantro
This is what probably led to the Chipotle following. Whichever way they do theirs, I found a way to create this rice online. Here you go.

> 1 cup cooked Jasmine rice
> 1 lime, juiced
> 1 tablespoon of lime zest
> ½ bunch of cilantro
> 1 tablespoon of coconut oil

Heat the wok and when it's hot, add the coconut oil around the top rim. Add the cooked rice and stir around for about 30 seconds. Add the cilantro, juice from the lime, and the zest and keep stirring. Stir for about 2 minutes until heated through and serve.[52]

Wild Rice Good For a Picnic
I also got this idea from the *Food52 Genius Recipes* cookbook and I'm going to fiddle with it a little more. Every time I want to start making this, it just looks too cumbersome but I've recreated this recipe so that I can do it. I'm all over it. It's so versatile and I can take this on a picnic like the name suggests. This was too good not to share.

> 1 cup cooked Jasmine rice
> ½ cup of cooked wild rice

---

52 I just saved a recipe online that included 1 tablespoon of lime zest that I wanted to mention. I'll have to try that next time.

2 celery stalks, chopped very small

1 bunch of green onions, chopped

1 tablespoon of white wine vinegar

1 tablespoon of olive oil

½ teaspoon of sea salt

Wild rice takes about 45 minutes as opposed to jasmine rice, which will take half the time. Make both and set aside. Chop the celery and green onions and toss into the combined rice. Blend white wine vinegar and olive oil and set aside. Mix cooked Jasmine rice and wild rice together. Mix the dressing in with green onions and celery and season with salt. Garnish with parsley leaves. How can this go wrong?

Fried Rice Staple

I make this all the time. Richard loves it and it's the quickest meal I can make with leftover steamed rice, carrots at the bottom of the veggie drawer, and peas in my freezer. You'll need a wok preferably, but if you don't have one, you can probably use a non-stick frying pan—your next best friend. If you're transitioning, you might even want to scramble an egg and toss it in there as well. I no longer do that. However, the world is your oyster with this one.

1 cup of steamed rice

½ cup of chopped onions

3 garlic cloves, smashed and minced

2 large carrots, diced or cut julienne style

½ bag frozen peas

2 tablespoons of organic gluten-free Tamari sauce

1 tablespoon of fish sauce (Okay to omit if you are committed to leaving out animal products.)

2 tablespoons of sesame oil

Heat your wok until it's hot. Add the sesame oil around the top of the wok so it drips down to the center. Add the onions, garlic, and carrots and let it simmer for about 2 minutes. Add the frozen peas and stir it around for another minute until everything looks softened. Add the rice, fish sauce, and Tamari sauce and consistently mix until heated through. Garnish with cilantro if desired and serve immediately.

Steamed Veggies

Another staple appliance to have in your kitchen is a steamer. You have to have a way to steam your vegetables all the time like you have a microwave to heat your food. I put cauliflower, carrots, asparagus, broccoli, and green beans (and even salmon when we cheat) in my steamer. I add garlic powder, sesame seeds, or onion powder right on my vegetables to bring out their taste and cover.

Roasted Vegetables

This is a no-brainer and quick fix as a side dish for anything you make. Vegetables are great to grill. I know you know this, but is it a habit to pull out the eggplant with bell peppers and grill these suckers as a side dish? We know this when we're at a BBQ or in a restaurant, but do we make these at home on a regular basis? Don't just bake your vegetables grill them. They're a lot more flavorful when grilled. I've also added roasted potatoes to them and baked everything right after and it was so pretty that I posted it all over social media. Good thing it tasted good too!

Eggplant

Carrots

Zucchini squash

Onions

Tomatoes

Chilies

Asparagus

Garlic

Lemon

Kale

Red, green, or yellow bell peppers

Green onions

Corn on the cob

Artichoke hearts, etc.

Cut vegetables in big pieces. Toss vegetables in a homemade salad dressing with vinegar, oil, and seasoning and set aside to marinate before putting them on the grill. Another way to season them is to lightly sprinkle garlic powder and olive oil with fresh herbs like diced marjoram, thyme, chives, or sage before grilling. Grilled vegetables make any dish look beautiful. Save fresh herbs to sprinkle on top when done too for a more advanced looking plate.

Sautéed Spinach with Garlic and Shitake Mushrooms

There is a right way and a wrong way to make this. If you make this the wrong way, you'll ruin any chances for your family to like this side dish and it's really delicious. I had this at a restaurant, most likely with a lot of butter, but I've improvised and swapped the butter for a healthier choice and we love it. You can add onions too, but we just like it with garlic.

1 bag of cleaned spinach[53]

1 box of Shitake mushrooms

2 tablespoons of coconut oil

5 big cloves of crushed and diced garlic

1 tablespoon of sherry for good measure

Heat the sauté pan until hot, but not burning hot. Add the coconut oil, the garlic, and the mushrooms. Sauté the garlic and mushrooms until the mushrooms become tender for about 3 minutes and add the sherry if desired. Add the entire bag of spinach into the frying pan, tossing the spinach consistently so that it doesn't burn and cooks thoroughly. Serve immediately.

---

53 You can go for the fresh bunch of spinach but remember to thoroughly clean the spinach because fresh spinach has a lot of dirt and has to be washed at least 3 times before being put in a bag ready for use. That's what the bag says anyway.

Mediterranean Cauliflower Sautéed in Lemon and Garlic

I got this from a Mediterranean restaurant and it was just delicious. I was curious enough to try the garlic cauliflower and, from that, I've made this a number of times. I might be missing a spice that turned the oil a bright yellow but it's still good. If you know what that spice is, you're lucky!

    1 cauliflower
    1 lemon
    5-6 garlic cloves or more
    5 tablespoons of olive oil
    Parsley, cilantro, tarragon, chives, or other favorite herb for garnish

Cut the cauliflower into small pieces. Steam the cauliflower for about 4 minutes until tender and a fork or knife easily pierces it. Remove and toss with 1 tablespoon of oil and lemon juice from about half the lemon. Heat non-stick frying pan until it gets hot. Add the oil and garlic and sauté for about 2 minutes. Add the cauliflower and let it cook until cauliflower has a nice brown look. Add the rest of the lemon juice and garnish with parsley.

Thanksgiving Sweet Potato Casserole

This is a favorite during Thanksgiving but why wait? I grew up on this dish with marshmallows roasted on top but my mother-in-law made this with a sugar and pecan topping and it was delicious. However, I would make this without the butter or marshmallows and add just a little brown sugar.

    3 sweet potatoes
    ½ cup of chopped pecans
    ¼ cup of brown sugar
    ¼ cup plant milk (Vanilla almond milk, preferably.
    1 tablespoon of molasses
    1 tablespoon of coconut oil

Cook the sweet potatoes in the oven at 400° for about an hour. They are done when they can be pierced easily with a knife. You can also cook them in the microwave for about 5-10 minutes, depending on size. Always pierce with a knife before cooking. Take out a casserole dish and line the sides with a little coconut oil. This will make cleaning easier and adds a taste of coconut too. Chop the walnuts and mix with brown sugar and set aside. Yes, brown sugar is granulated sugar with molasses, but you can either add more sugar or just add molasses (I add molasses). Mix the pecans with the sugar and set aside. (If you like the taste of sweet yams, you don't even really need sugar.) Peel the yams when they are cooked and smash them with the milk, adding gradually, with a bean masher. It's okay if they are lumpy. Drizzle the molasses on top and then add the sugar and walnuts. Reduce the oven to 350° and bake for about 20 minutes until the molasses underneath has soaked through.

DESSERT

Homemade Plant-Based Ice Cream

As soon as I can figure out what is wrong with my ice cream maker, I'm going to try coconut milk, vanilla almond milk, an egg replacer, and vanilla with a little sugar. This will take some tweaking and some time, but the last time I made ice cream, my ice cream maker didn't seem to be working. If you have an ice cream maker that has been sitting in your garage, you're in luck! I got mine from my mother-in-law's garage. She knew I liked to cook and gave it to me like getting rid of an old pair of shoes. Little did she know how much I would use it because we love homemade ice cream. I took homemade ice cream to a 4th of July BBQ and served it with fresh raspberries and blueberries and, boy, was it was hit!

Banana Nut Bread

I buy gluten-free chocolate banana bread at a gluten-free bakery. There is no need to have this with whole-wheat flour. This bread can be made using applesauce, chocolate, nuts, and real fresh bananas. It can be made purely vegan and be just as good, if not better, than regular banana nut bread. I'm not much of a baker but if you are, send me a good recipe and I'll try it.

Sweet Staple

I have gotten used to buying berries all the time. They're good for smoothies, which was practically the only reason I bought them, but they make for a great dessert. I actually found a brand new can of whipped cream at the bottom of my fridge door and was happy to have it with some strawberries. I live in southern California so strawberries are in season practically all year round but they're at their peak during March and April. I buy blueberries, raspberries, and even blackberries. I sauté them, have them with whipped cream, with chocolate, in a salad, for breakfast, in a fruit bowl, as a snack, as a topping, and soon in a cocktail. It's my sweet staple.

Sticky Rice

My friend makes sticky rice all the time and I went looking for it. I bought some and will create an Asian dessert with mango I love to have in a restaurant. Actually, I'll make this now.

About the Author

As an owner and operator of The Sonoma Wine Nest, a Vacation Rental in Sonoma County, I currently operate this business from home in Los Angeles. I also own a small business helping other small business owners expand their services. From short-term rentals to Silicon Valley's technology firms, I have managed anything from housekeeping to online marketing to various other projects that can be done from home. As I submit the final draft for this manuscript, I have just recently accepted an Independent Sales position with Getty Images that I can also work from home. I agree with my dad that I now consider this role my sweet spot. All images on my website and on my blogs are my own and can be found at SonomaWineNest.com and ClaudiaCastro.com.

While working full time at The Orange County Register, I acquired a bachelor's degree in creative writing. After completing college, I moved to Los Angeles from Orange County and held a position at New York Cablevision's satellite office for TV ad sales and then Showtime Networks before moving to New York selling billboard ads with Vista Media. After holding several media roles in sales and marketing I moved back to Los Angeles and attained a real estate license. After working as a licensed mortgage consultant, I held various roles in property management but was still in search of a career in writing. After nearly 25 years in sales and marketing from media sales to real estate, I was fortunate to launch Sonoma Wine Nest LLC and start a small home business that enables me to continue my pursuit for writing.

I have always been passionate about writing and now after many roles from Los Angeles to New York, I can share many lessons I've learned on this journey of finding work that is fulfilling.

My latest experiment with diet is one that has interested me a lot. I've been a member of at least 15 different gyms, have sold nutritional products on the side and have always been concerned with my health. When I finally gathered the courage to submit my manuscript to a publisher just for feedback, it was accepted and fulfilled a lifelong dream.

Happily married to Richard who I moved back to Los Angeles to marry, we attend a church that keeps us busy whether it's teaching Sunday class or leading a family group. Richard and I also love to frequently visit our home in Northern California to constantly make home improvements for our guests like in the backyard but often take a break for wine tastings in between.

A free eBook edition is available with the purchase of this book.

To claim your free eBook edition:

1. Download the Shelfie app.
2. Write your name in upper case in the box.
3. Use the Shelfie app to submit a photo.
4. Download your eBook to any device.

Shelfie

A **free** eBook edition is available
with the purchase of this print book.

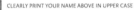

CLEARLY PRINT YOUR NAME ABOVE IN UPPER CASE

Instructions to claim your free eBook edition:
1. Download the Shelfie app for Android or iOS
2. Write your name in **UPPER CASE** above
3. Use the Shelfie app to submit a photo
4. Download your eBook to any device

Print & Digital Together Forever.

Snap a photo

Free eBook

Read anywhere

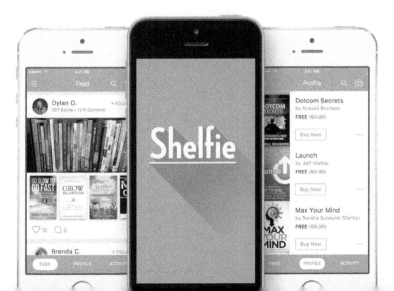

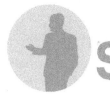

The Morgan James
Speakers Group

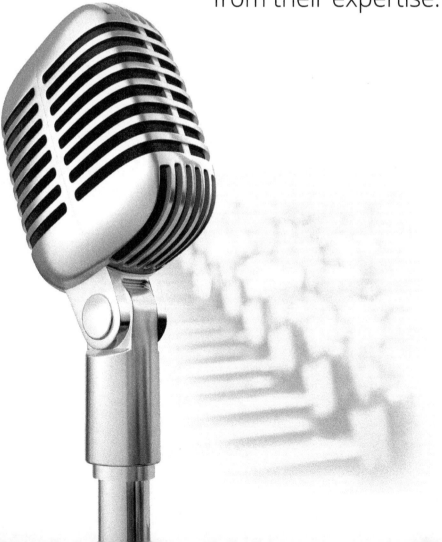

🡕 www.TheMorganJamesSpeakersGroup.com

We connect Morgan James published
authors with live and online events
and audiences whom will benefit
from their expertise.